Medical **Spanish** in **Pediatrics**

Medical **Spanish** in **Pediatrics**

AN **INSTANT** TRANSLATOR

Isam Nasr, MD, FACEP
Department of Emergency Medicine
Cook County Hospital
Chicago, Illinois

Marco A. Cordero, MD, FACEP
Department of Emergency Medicine
Palos Community Hospital
Palos Heights, Illinois

Foreword by David F. Soglin, MD, FAAP
Department of Pediatrics
Cook County Hospital
Chicago, Illinois

Saunders
An Imprint of Elsevier

SAUNDERS
An Imprint of Elsevier

The Curtis Center
Independence Square West
Philadelphia, Pennsylvania 19106

Medical Spanish In Pediatrics:
An Instant Translator   ISBN 0–7216–8447–5

Library of Congress Cataloging-in-Publication Data

Nasr, Isam
    Medical Spanish in pediatrics: an instant translator / Isam
        Nasr, Marco Cordero.—1st ed.
      p. : cm.
    ISBN 0–7216–8447–5
      1. Spanish language—Conversation and phrase books
(for medical personnel). 2. Pediatrics—Terminology.
I. Cordero, Marco. II. Title.
    PC4120.M3 N39 2000
    468.3′421′02461—dc21   00-026970

Editor-in-Chief: Lisette Bralow
Acquisitions Editor: Stephanie Donley
Project Manager: Mary Anne Folcher
Production Manager: Frank Polizzano
Book Designer: Gene Harris
Indexer: Dennis Dolan

Printed in the United States of America

Last digit is the print number: 9   8   7   6   5   4   3

To Our Families

Foreword

I know of no other book that is as immediately useful for taking care of pediatric patients from Spanish-speaking families as this one. The authors previously developed and published a medical Spanish pocket manual that has allowed nonSpanish–speaking physicians to communicate with exclusively Spanish speaking–patients. Now these physicians have added this text designed for use with pediatric patients. Drs. Nasr and Cordero have taught our pediatric residents Spanish. Many are able to communicate effectively with Spanish speaking–patients after only a few sessions. This text has thus been used extensively in our pediatric emergency department for over a year.

Medical Spanish in Pediatrics: An Instant Translator has been designed for practical use. From clear explanations of pronunciation, through anatomical terms, to chapters organized by presenting complaint, the authors have kept in mind busy physicians trying to communicate with their patients and caregivers. They start with such common-sense phrases as "Is there someone with you who speaks English?" and "Please speak slowly." They continue to the common questions one would ask for each of the most common presenting complaints.

Each chapter includes practical instructions for performing the physical examination, such as "Breathe deeply" as well as phrases designed to describe the likely work-up.

Common discharge instructions are included for each complaint. Without prior knowledge of Spanish, the physician using this text will be able to instruct parents on how to give medicine, what follow-up is needed, and what the indications are for a return visit. The questions and phrases in each chapter were designed through the authors' own experiences of taking care of children with input from practicing pediatricians and pediatric emergency medicine physicians. Each question is presented in English and Spanish with the Spanish pronunciation shown.

This is truly a rare English-Spanish manual. There is no

need to look up individual words or to have prior knowledge of Spanish to use it. Designed by practicing emergency medicine physicians, this book is practical. As a severely language-impaired physician, even I am able to work independently with most Spanish speaking–families. It belongs in the pocket or library of every physician who treats Spanish speaking–pediatric patients.

David F. Soglin, MD
Department of Pediatrics
Cook County Hospital
Chicago, Illinois

Preface

Caring for the ill child poses many challenges even for the most experienced physician. Delivery of care may be compromised owing to language barriers between health care workers and guardians of the child. With the increasing numbers of non-English–speaking Latinos living in the United States today, it becomes essential that health care providers familiarize themselves with certain sentences and phrases in Spanish in order to improve dialogue with patients and their families.

The purpose of *Medical Spanish in Pediatrics: An Instant Translator* is to facilitate communication between healthcare workers and their patients who speak only Spanish. The book is divided into several chapters based on presenting pediatric complaints, such as fever, vomiting, and abdominal pain, among others. Each chapter consists of a series of questions pertaining to the complaint. Most questions require a simple Yes or No answer from the patients, parents, or caregivers. Each question or phrase has the exact Spanish translation next to it—with common terms and phrases that are needed during the physical examination and for explaining diagnoses, work-up plans, and dispositions. Discharge instructions specific to each complaint are also included.

Minimal or no knowledge of the Spanish language is necessary for the healthcare professional to utilize this text successfully. Physicians, nurses, medical students, paramedics, physician assistants, and medical technicians will find the manual ideal for use in their practices, emergency departments, out-patient clinics, and hospital units. Although it may be used to obtain pertinent information from Spanish speaking–persons, *Medical Spanish in Pediatrics: An Instant Translator* should not be considered a substitute for the skill and experience of a bilingual health care professional.

Acknowledgment

We would like to thank
Drs. José M. Rodriguez and David Soglin
for their help with this project.

Contents

Introduction

Anatomy

Abdomen	El abdomen Ehl ab-**doh**-mehn	Buttock	La nalga La **nahl**-gah
Ankle	El tobillo Ehl toh-**bee**-yhoh	Calf	La pantorilla Lah pahn-toh-**ree**-yhah
Anus	El ano El **ah**-noh	Cervix	El cuello uterino Ehl **kweh**-yoh oo-teh-**ree**-noh
Appendix	El apéndice Ehl ah-**pehn**-dee-seh		
Arm	El brazo Ehl **brah**-soh	Cheek	La mejilla Lah meh-**hee**-yhah
Artery	La arteria Lah ahr-**teh**-ree-ah	Chest	El pecho Ehl **peh**-choh
Axilla	La axila Lah ag-**see**-lah	Chin	El mentón Ehl mehn-**tohn**
Back	La espalda Lah ehs-**pahl**-dah	Clavicle	La clavícula Lah klah-**vee**-koo-lah
Bladder	La vejiga Lah beh-**hee**-gah	Ear	El oído / La oreja Ehl oh-**ee**-doh / Lah oh-**reh**-ha
Body	El cuerpo Ehl **kwehr**-poh		
Bone	El hueso Ehl **weh**-soh	Elbow	El codo Ehl **koh**-doh
Brain	El cerebro Ehl seh-**reh**-broh	Eye	El ojo Ehl **oh**-hoh
Breasts	Los senos Lohs **seh**-nohs	Eyebrow	La ceja Lah **seh**-hah
		Eyelash	La pestaña Lah pehs-**tah**-nyah

Eyelid	El párpado Ehl **pahr**-pah-doh	Head	La cabeza Lah kah-**beh**-sah
Face	La cara Lah **kah**-rah	Heart	El corazón Ehl koh-rah-**sohn**
Finger	El dedo Ehl **deh**-doh	Heel	El talón Ehl tah-**lohn**
Fingernail	La uña Lah **oo**-nyah	Hip	La cadera Lah kah-**deh**-rah
Foot	El pie Ehl pee-eh	Intestines	Los intestinos Lohs **een**-tehs-**tee**-nohs
Fontanelle	La mollera / La fontanela Lah moh-**yeh**-rah / lah fohn-tah-**neh**-lah	Joint	La articula-ción Lah ahr-tee-koo-lah-**see-ohn**
Forearm	El antebrazo Ehl ahn-teh-**brah**-soh	Kidney	El riñón Ehl ree-**nyohn**
Forehead	La frente Lah **frehn**-teh	Knee	La rodilla Lah roh-**dee**-yhah
Foreskin	El prepucio Ehl preh-**poo**-see-oh	Knuckle	El nudillo Ehl noo-**dee**-yoh
Gallbladder	La vesícula biliar Lah beh-**see**-koo-lah bee-lee-**ahr**	Larynx	La laringe Lah lah-**reen**-heh
Gingiva / gums	Las encías Lahs ehn-**see**-ahs	Leg	La pierna Lah **pee-ehr**-nah
Groin	La ingle Lah **een**-gleh	Lips	Los labios Lohs **lah**-bee-ohs
Hair	El pelo / El cabello Ehl **peh**-loh / Ehl kah-**beh**-yoh	Liver	El hígado Ehl **ee**-gah-doh
Hand	La mano Lah **mah**-noh		

Lung	El pulmón Ehl pool-**mohn**	Prostate	La próstata Lah **prohs**-tah-tah
Lymph node	El ganglio linfático Ehl gahn-glee-oh leen-**fah**-tee-koh	Pupil	La pupila Lah poo-**pee**-lah
		Rectum	El recto Ehl **reg**-toh
Mandible	La mandíbula Lah mahn-**dee-hoo**-lah	Rib	La costilla Lah kohs-**tee**-yah
Mouth	La boca Lah **boh**-kah	Scalp	El cuero ca-belludo Ehl **kweh**-roh kah-beh-**yuh**-doh
Muscle	El músculo Ehl **moos**-koo-loh		
Navel	El ombligo Ehl ohm-**blee**-goh	Scapula	La escápula Lah ehs-**kah**-poo-lah
Neck	El cuello Ehl **kweh**-yoh	Scrotum	El escroto Ehl ehs-**kroh**-toh
Nerve	El nervio Ehl **nehr**-bee-oh	Shoulder	El hombro Ehl **ohm**-broh
Nipple	El pezón Ehl peh-**sohn**	Skin	La piel Lah pee-ehl
Nose	La nariz Lah nah-**rees**	Skull	El cráneo Ehl **krah**-neh-oh
Ovary	El ovario Ehl oh-**bah**-ree-oh	Spine	El espinazo Ehl ehs-pee-**nah**-soh
Pancreas	El páncreas Ehl **pahn**-kreh-ahs	Spleen	El bazo Ehl **bah**-soh
Pelvis	La pelvis Lah **pehl**-bees	Sternum	El esternón Ehl ehs-tehr-**nohn**
Penis	El pene Ehl **peh**-neh	Stomach	El estómago Ehl ehs-**toh**-mah-goh

Tendon	El tendón Ehl tehn-**dohn**	Tubes	Los tubos Lohs **too**-bohs
Testicles	Los testículos Lohs tehs-**tee-koo**-lohs	Umbilical cord	El cordón umbilical Ehl kohr-**dohn** oom-bee-le-**kahl**
Thigh	El muslo Ehl **moos**-loh		
Thorax	El tórax Ehl **toh**-raks	Urethra	La uretra Lah oo-**reh**-trah
Throat	La garganta Lah gahr-**gahn**-tah		
Thumb	El pulgar Ehl pool-**gahr**	Uterus	El útero / La matriz Ehl **oo**-teh-roh / Lah mah-**trees**
Thymus	El timo Ehl **tee**-moh		
Thyroid	La tiroides Lah tee-roh-ee-dehs	Uvula	La campanilla Lah kahm-pah-**nee**-yah
Toes	Los dedos de los pies Lohs **deh**-dohs deh lohs pee-ehs	Vagina	La vagina Lah bah-**hee**-nah
		Vein	La vena Lah **beh**-nah
Tongue	La lengua Lah **lehn**-gwah	Vocal cords	Las cuerdas vocales Lahs **kwehr**-dahs boh-**kah**-lehs
Tonsils	Las anginas Lahs ahn-**hee**-nahs		
Tooth	El diente Ehl dee-**ehn**-teh	Waist	La cintura Lah seen-**too**-rah
Trachea	La tráquea Lah **trah**-keh-ah	Wrist	La muñeca Lah moo-**nyeh**-kah

Common Terms

I speak a little Spanish.		Hablo un poco de Español. **Ah**-bloh oon poh-koh deh Ehs-pah-**nyohl.**	
Please answer *yes* or *no*.		Por favor, conteste *si* o *no*. Pohr fah-**bohr** kohn-**tehs**-teh ooo oh noh.	
Please speak slowly.		Por favor, hable despacio. Pohr fah-bohr **ah**-bleh dehs-**pah**-see-oh.	
Hello.		Hola. **Oh**-lah.	
I	Yo Yoh	They	Ellos / Ellas Eh-yohs / Eh-yahs
He	Él Ehl	We (*masculine*)	Nosotros Noh-**soh**-trohs
She	Ella Eh-yah	We (*feminine*)	Nosotras Noh-**soh**-trahs
You (*familiar*)	Tú Too	You (*formal*)	Usted Oos-**tehd**
		You (*formal plural*)	Ustedes Oos-**teh**-dehs
I am the doctor (*male*) . . .		Soy el doctor . . . Soy ehl dohk-**tohr** . . .	
I am the doctor (*female*) . . .		Soy la doctora . . . Soy lah dohk-**toh**-rah . . .	

I am the nurse . . .	Soy la enfermera / el enfermero . . . Soy lah ehn-fehr-**meh**-rah / ehl ehn-fehr-**meh**-roh . . .
How are you?	¿Cómo está usted? **Koh**-moh ehs-**tah** oos-**tehd?**
How do you feel?	¿Cómo se siente? **Koh**-moh seh **see-ehn**-teh?
Good morning.	Buenos días. **Bweh**-nohs **dee**-ahs.
Good afternoon.	Buenas tardes. **Bweh**-nahs **tahr**-dehs.
Good evening / night.	Buenas noches. **Bweh**-nahs **noh**-chehs.
What is your name?	¿Cuál es su nombre? **Kwahl** ehs soo **nohm**-breh?
	¿Cómo se llama? **Koh**-moh seh **yah**-mah?
What is your last name?	¿Cuál es su apellido? **Kwahl** ehs soo ah-peh-**yee**-doh?
What is the baby's name?	¿Cuál es el nombre del bebé? **Kwahl** ehs ehl **nohm**-breh dehl beh-**beh?**
What is the child's name?	¿Cuál es el nombre del niño / de la niña? **Kwahl** ehs ehl-**nohm**-breh dehl **nee**-nyoh / deh lah **nee**-nyah?

Does he / she have your last name?	¿Él / Ella tiene el mismo apellido como usted? Ehl / eh-yah **tee-eh**-neh ehl **mees**-moh ah-peh-**yee**-doh **koh**-moh oos-**tehd?**
How old (in years) is he / she?	¿Cuántos años tiene él / ella? **Kwahn**-tohs **ah**-nyohs **tee-eh**-neh ehl / eh-yah?
How old (in months) is he / she?	¿Cuántos meses tiene él / ella? **Kwahn**-tohs **meh**-sehs **tee-eh**-neh ehl / eh-yah?
How old (in weeks) is he / she?	¿Cuántas semanas tiene él / ella? **Kwahn**-tahs seh-**mah**-nahs **tee-eh**-neh ehl / eh-yah?
What is his / her date of birth?	¿Cuál es su fecha de nacimiento? **Kwahl** ehs soo **feh**-chah deh nah-see-mee-**ehn**-toh?
___ month	___ mes mehs
___ day	___ día **dee**-ah
___ year	___ año **ah**-nyoh
What is the problem?	¿Cuál es el problema? **Kwahl** ehs ehl proh-**bleh**-mah?
Does your child have allergies?	¿Tiene alergias su niño / niña? **Tee-eh**-neh ah-**lehr**-hee-ahs soo **nee**-nyoh / **nee**-nyah?

Is he / she allergic to penicillin?

¿Es alérgico (a) a la penicilina?
Ehs ah-**lehr**-hee-koh (ah) ah
lah peh-nee-see-**lee**-nah?

Lie down.

Acuéstese.
Ah-**kwehs**-teh-seh.

Lie the baby down.

Acuéste al bebé.
Ah-**kwehs**-teh ahl beh-**beh.**

Lie him / her down.

Acuéstelo / acuéstela.
Ah-**kwehs**-teh-loh / ah-**kwehs**-teh-lah.

Get up.

Levántese.
Leh-**bahn**-teh-seh.

Get him / her up.

Levántelo / levántela.
Leh-**bahn**-teh-loh / leh-**bahn**-teh-lah.

Stand up.

Párese.
Pah-reh-seh.

Stand him / her up.

Párelo / párela.
Pah-reh-loh / **pah**-reh-lah.

Sit down.

Siéntese.
See-ehn-teh-seh.

Sit him / her down.

Siéntelo / siéntela.
See-ehn-teh-loh / **see-ehn**-teh-lah.

Turn around.

Voltéese.
Bohl-**teh-eh**-seh.

Turn him / her around.

Voltéelo/voltéela.
Bohl-**teh-eh**-loh / bohl-**teh-eh**-lah.

Turn on your right side.	Voltéese al lado derecho. Bohl-**teh-eh**-seh ahl **lah**-doh deh-**reh**-choh.
Turn on your left side.	Voltéese al lado izquierdo. Bohl-**teh-eh**-seh ahl **lah**-doh ees-**kee-ehr**-doh.
Lie on your back.	Acuéstese boca arriba. Ah-**kwehs**-teh-seh **boh**-kah ah- **rhee**-bah.
Lie on your stomach.	Acuéstese boca abajo. Ah-**kwehs**-teh-seh **boh**-kah ah- **bah**-hoh.
Relax, please.	Por favor, relájese. Pohr fah-**bohr** reh-**lah**-heh-seh.
Calm down.	Cálmese. **Kahl**-meh-seh.
Please, don't move.	Por favor, no se mueva. Pohr fah-**bohr** noh seh **mweh**- bah.
Do not be afraid.	No tenga miedo. Noh tehn-gah mee-eh-doh.
Take a deep breath.	Respire profundo. Rhes-**pee**-reh proh-**foon**-doh.
Show me.	Enséñeme / muéstrame. Ehn-**seh**-nyeh-meh/ moo-**ehs**- trah-meh.
What?	¿Qué? **Keh?**

Who?	¿Quién?
	Kee-**ehn?**
Where?	¿Dónde?
	Dohn-deh?
Why?	¿Por qué?
	Pohr-**keh?**
Because	Por que
	Pohr-**keh**
How?	¿Cómo?
	Koh-moh?
Which?	¿Cuál?
	Kwahl?
When?	¿Cuándo?
	Kwahn-doh?
To where?	¿A dónde?
	Ah **dohn**-deh?
For how long?	¿Por cuánto tiempo?
	Pohr **kwahn**-toh **tee-ehm**-poh?
Since when?	¿Desde cuándo?
	Dehs-deh **kwahn**-doh?
How long ago?	¿Hace cuánto tiempo?
	Ah-seh **kwahn**-toh **tee-ehm**-poh?
How often?	¿Con qué frecúencia?
	Kohn **keh** freh-**kwehn**-see-ah?
How much?	¿Cuánto?
	Kwahn-toh?

Here	Aquí / acá Ah-**kee** / ah-**kah**
There	Allí / allá Ah-**yee** / ah-**yah**
This	Este Ehs-teh
That	Ese Eh-seh
During	Durante Doo-**rahn-**teh
Take off your clothes.	Quítese la ropa. **Kee**-teh-seh lah **roh**-pah.
Take off his / her clothes / diaper.	Quítele la ropa / el pañal. **Kee**-teh-leh lah **roh**-pah / ehl pah-**nyahl.**
Put on his / her clothes / diaper.	Póngale la ropa / el pañal. **Pohn**-gah-leh lah **roh**-pah / ehl pah-**nyahl.**
He / she needs stitches.	Él / ella necesita puntadas / suturas. Ehl / eh-yah neh-seh-**see**-tah poon-**tah**-dahs / soo-**too**-rahs.
He / she needs an operation.	Él / ella necesita una operación. Ehl / eh-yah neh-seh-**see**-tah **oo**-nah oh-peh-rah-**see-ohn.**
He / she needs an injection.	Él / ella necesita una inyección. Ehl / eh-yah neh-seh-**see**-tah **oo**-nah een-jeg-**see-ohn.**

He / she needs to take medication.	Él / ella necesita tomar medicina. Ehl / eh-yah neh-seh-**see**-tah toh-**mahr** meh-dee-**see**-nah.
He / she needs to return here.	Él / ella necesita regresar aquí. Ehl / eh-yah neh-seh-**see**-tah reh-greh-**sahr** ah-**kee**.
He / she needs blood tests.	Él / ella necesita análisis de sangre. Ehl / eh-yah neh-seh-**see**-tah ah-**nah**-lee-sees deh **sahn**-greh.
He / she needs an X-ray.	Él / ella necesita una radiografía / rayos X. Ehl / eh-yah neh-seh-**see**-tah **oo**-nah **rah**-dee-oh-grah-**fee**-**ah** / **rah**-yhohs **eh**-keys.
We need to admit him / her.	Necesitamos internarlo (a) / admitirlo (a). Neh-seh-see-**tah**-mohs **een**-tehr-**nahr**-loh / ad-mee-**teer**-loh.
He / she needs a cast.	Él / ella necesita yeso. Ehl / eh-yah neh-seh-**see**-tah **yeh**-soh.
He / she needs to see a specialist.	Él / ella necesita ver a un especialista. Ehl / eh-yah neh-seh-**see**-tah behr ah oon ehs-**peh-see**-ah-lees-tah.
He / she needs an ultrasound.	Él / ella necesita un ultrasonido. Ehl / eh-yah neh-seh-**see**-tah oon **ool**-trah-soh-**nee**-doh.

He / she needs a urine test.

Él / ella necesita una prueba de orina.
Ehl / eh-yah neh-seh-**see**-tah **oo**-nah **proo-eh**-bah deh oh-**ree**-nah.

He / she needs a Foley catheter.

Él / ella necesita una sonda.
Ehl / eh-yah neh-seh-**see**-tah **oo**-nah **sohn**-dah.

I need to examine him / her.

Necesito examinarlo / la.
Neh-seh-**see**-toh eg-sah-mee-**nahr**-loh / lah.

I need to examine his / her . . .

Necesito examinar su . . .
Neh seh-**see**-toh eg sah-mee-**nahr** soo . . .

I need to examine him for a hernia.

Necesito examinarlo para ver si tiene una hernia.
Neh-seh-**see**-toh eg-sah-mee-**nahr**-loh pah-rah behr see **tee-eh**-neh **oo**-nah **ehr**-nee-ah.

Turn your head and cough.

Voltée la cabeza y tosa.
Bohl-**teh**-eh lah kah-**beh**-sah ee **toh**-sah.

He / she needs intravenous fluid.

Él / ella necesita suero intravenoso.
Ehl / eh-yah neh-seh-**see**-tah soo-eh-roh / een-trah-beh-**noh**-soh.

He / she has an infection.

Él / ella tiene una infección.
Ehl / eh-yah **tee-eh**-neh **oo**-nah een-feg-**see-ohn.**

He / she has a fracture.

Él / ella tiene una fractura.
Ehl / eh-yah **tee-eh**-neh **oo**-nah frag-**too**-rah.

He / she has a sprain.

Él / ella tiene una torcedura.
Ehl / eh-yah **tee-eh**-neh **oo**-nah tohr-seh-**doo**-rah.

He / she has pneumonia.

Él / ella tiene pulmonía.
Ehl / eh-yah **tee-eh**-neh pool-moh-**nee**-ah.

It is necessary.

Es necesario.
Ehs neh-seh-**sah**-ree-oh.

It is important.

Es importante.
Ehs eem-pohr-**tahn**-teh.

It is better.

Es mejor.
Ehs meh-**hohr.**

It is worse.

Es peor.
Ehs peh-**ohr.**

It is the same.

Es igual.
Ehs ee-**gwahl.**

It is a lot.

Es mucho.
Ehs **moo**-choh.

It is a little.

Es poco.
Ehs **poh**-koh.

It is sufficient / enough.

Es suficiente.
Ehs soo-fee-see-**ehn**-teh.

It is hard.

Está duro.
Ehs-tah **doo**-roh.

It is soft.

Está suave.
Ehs-tah soo-**ah**-beh.

He / she / it / is big.

Está grande.
Ehs-tah **grahn**-deh.

He / she / it / is small.

Está pequeño (a).
Ehs-tah peh-**keh**-nyoh (ah).

It is cold.

Está frío.
Ehs-tah **free**-oh.

It is hot.

Está caliente.
Ehs-tah kah-lee-**ehn**-teh.

It is lukewarm.

Está tibio (a).
Ehs-**tah too** boo-oh (ah).

He / she / it / is tall.

Es alto (a).
Ehs **ahl**-toh (ah).

He / she / it / is short.

Es bajo (a).
Ehs **bah**-hoh (ah).

He / she / it / is okay.

Está bien.
Ehs-**tah** bee-ehn.

He / she / it / is bad.

Está mal.
Ehs-**tah** mahl.

He / she is happy.

Está alegre.
Ehs-**tah** ah-**leh**-greh.

He / she is sad.

Está triste.
Ehs-**tah trees**-teh.

Miscellaneous Terms

Appointment	Cita **See**-tah	Pill	Píldora / pastilla **Peel**-doh-rah pahs-**tee**- yhah
To admit	Internar **Een**-tehr-**nahr**	Tablet	Tableta Tah-**bleh**-tah

To discharge	Dar de alta Dahr deh **ahl**-tah	Capsule	Cápsula **Kap**-soo-lah
Blood	Sangre **Sahn**-greh	Injection	Inyección Een-jeg-**see-ohn**
Urine	Orina Oh-**ree**-nah	Ointment	Pomada Poh-**mah**-dah
Saliva	Saliva Sah-**lee**-bah	Lotion	Loción Loh-**see-ohn**
Blood clot	Coágulo de sangre Koh-**ah**-goo-loh deh **sahn**-greh	Swollen	Hinchado Een-**chah**-doh
Vomit	Vómito **Boh**-mee-toh	Bruise	Moretón Moh-reh-**tohn**
Fever	Fiebre **Fee-eh**-breh	Dizzy	Mareada (o) Mah-reh-**ah**-dah (oh)
Feces	Heces **Eh**-sehs	Dizziness	Mareos Mah-**reh**-ohs
Phlegm	Flema **Fleh**-mah	Numb	Entumido (a) Ehn-too-**mee**-doh (ah)
Mucus	Mocosidad Moh-koh-see-**dahd**	Fracture	Fractura Frag-**too**-rah

Sweat	Sudor Soo-**dohr**	Sprain	Torcedura Tohr-seh-**doo**-rah
Tears	Lágrimas **Lah**-gree-mahs	Faint	Desmayo Dehs-**mah**-yhoh
Discharge	Deshecho Dehs-**eh**-choh	Pain	Dolor Doh-**lohr**
Burning	Ardor Ahr-**dohr**	Itching	Comezón Koh-meh-**sohn**
Cramps	Calambres Kah-**lahm**-brehs	Chills	Escalofríos Ehs-kah-loh-**free-ohs**
Rash	Salpullido Sahl-poo-**yee**-doh	Blisters	Ampollas Ahm-**poh**-yahs
Scratch	Rascar Rahs-**kahr**	Burn	Quemadura Keh-mah-**doo**-rah

Colors

White	Blanco **Blahn**-koh	Green	Verde **Behr**-deh
Red	Rojo **Roh**-ho	Purple	Morado Moh-**rah**-doh
Yellow	Amarillo Ah-mah-**ree**-yoh	Gray	Gris Grees

Brown	Café	Black	Negro
	Kah-**feh**		**Neh**-groh
Blue	Azul	Pink	Rosa
	ah-**sool**		**Roh**-sah

Time

Today	Hoy	Oy
Yesterday	Ayer	Ah-**yehr**
Day before yesterday	Ante ayer	Ahn-teh ah-**yehr**
Tomorrow	Mañana	Mah-**nyah**-nah
Day after tomorrow	Pasado mañana	Pah-**sah**-doh mah-**nyah**-nah
Week	Semana	Seh-**mah**-nah
Next week	Próxima semana	**Prog**-see-mah seh-**mah**-nah
Last week	Semana pasada	Seh-**mah**-nah pah-**sah**-dah
Month	Mes	Mehs
Year	Año	**Ah**-nyoh

Days of the week

Monday	Lunes	**Loo**-nehs
Tuesday	Martes	**Mahr**-tehs
Wednesday	Miércoles	**Mee-ehr**-koh-lehs
Thursday	Jueves	**Hweh**-behs

Friday	Viernes	**Bee-ehr**-nehs
Saturday	Sabado	**Sah**-bah-doh
Sunday	Domingo	Doh-**meen**-goh

Months

January	Enero	Eh-**neh**-roh
February	Febrero	Feh-**breh**-roh
March	Marzo	**Mahr**-soh
April	Abril	Ah-**breel**
May	Mayo	**Mah**-yoh
June	Junio	**Hoo**-nee-oh
July	Julio	**Hoo**-lee-oh
August	Agosto	Ah-**gohs**-toh
September	Septiembre	Sep-**tee-ehm**-breh
October	Octubre	Og-**too**-breh
November	Noviembre	Noh-**bee-ehm**-breh
December	Diciembre	Dee-**see-ehm**-breh

Cardinal Numbers

| Zero | Cero | **Seh**-roh |
| One | Uno | **Oo**-noh |

Two	Dos	Dohs
Three	Tres	Trehs
Four	Cuatro	**Kwah**-troh
Five	Cinco	**Seen**-koh
Six	Seis	Says
Seven	Siete	**See-eh**-teh
Eight	Ocho	**Oh**-choh
Nine	Nueve	**Nweh**-beh
Ten	Diez	Dee-ehs
Eleven	Once	**Ohn**-seh
Twelve	Doce	**Doh**-seh
Thirteen	Trece	**Treh**-seh
Fourteen	Catorce	Kah-**tohr**-seh
Fifteen	Quince	**Keen**-seh
Sixteen	Dieciseis	**Dee-eh**-see-says
Seventeen	Diecisiete	**Dee-eh**-see-**see-eh**-teh
Eighteen	Dieci-ocho	**Dee-eh**-see-**oh**-choh
Nineteen	Dieci-nueve	**Dee-eh**-see-**nweh**-beh
Twenty	Veinte	**Bein**-teh

Twenty one	Vein-tiuno	**Bein**-tee-**oo**-noh
Twenty two	Veintidos	**Bein**-tee-dohs
Thirty	Treinta	**Treh-een**-tah
Forty	Cuarenta	Kwah-**rehn**-tah
Fifty	Cin-cuenta	Seen-**kwehn**-tah
Sixty	Sesenta	Seh-**sehn**-tah
Seventy	Setenta	Seh-**tehn**-tah
Eighty	Ochenta	Oh-**chehn**-tah
Ninety	Noventa	Noh-**behn**-tah
One Hundred	Cien	See-**ehn**
One Thousand	Mil	Meel

Pediatric Patient Registration

Registración del paciente pediátrico

Reh-hees-trah-**see-ohn** dehl pah-see-**ehn**-teh peh-dee-**ah**-tree-koh

What is the child's name?

¿Cómo se llama el niño / la niña?
Koh-moh seh **yah**-mah ehl **nee**-nyoh / lah **nee**-nyah?

What is the child's last name?

¿Cuál es el apellido del niño / la niña?
Kwahl ehs ehl ah-peh-**yee**-doh dehl **nee**-nyoh / lah **nee**-nyah?

What is the child's birthdate?

¿Cuál es la fecha de nacimiento del niño / la niña?
Kwahl ehs lah **feh**-chah deh nah-see-mee-**ehn**-toh dehl **nee**-nyoh / lah **nee**-nyah?

How old is the child?

¿Cuántos años tiene el niño / la niña?
Kwahn-tohs ah-nyohs **tee-eh**-neh ehl **nee**-nyoh / lah **nee**-nyah?

What is the child's social security number?

¿Cuál es el número de seguro social del niño / la niña?
Kwahl ehs ehl **noo**-meh-roh deh seh-**goo**-roh soh-see-ahl dehl **nee**-nyoh / lah **nee**-nyah?

What is your relationship to the child?

¿Cuál es su relación con el niño / la niña?
Kwahl ehs soo reh-lah-**see-ohn** kohn ehl **nee**-nyoh / la **nee**-nyah?

What is your name?

¿Cómo se llama usted?
Koh-moh seh **yah**-mah oos-**tehd**?

What is your last name?

¿Cuál es su apellido?
Kwahl ehs soo ah-peh-**yee**-doh?

What is your address?

¿Cuál es su dirección?
Kwahl ehs soo dee-reg-**see-ohn**?

What is your telephone number?

¿Cuál es su número de teléfono?
Kwahl ehs soo **noo**-meh-roh deh teh-**leh**-foh-noh?

Are you . . . ?	¿Es usted . . . ? Ehs oos-**tehd** . . . ?
__ married	__ casado (a) kah-**sah**-doh (ah)
__ single	__ soltero (a) sol-**teh**-roh (ah)
__ widowed	__ viudo (a) bee-**oo**-doh (ah)
__ divorced	__ divorciado (a) dee-bohr-**see-ah**-doh (ah)
__ separated	__ separado (a) seh-pah-**rah**-doh (ah)

Do you speak English?	¿Habla usted Inglés? **Ah**-blah oos-**tehd** Een-**glehs?**
Is there someone with you who speaks English?	¿Hay alguien con usted que hable Inglés? Eye **ahl**-gee-ehn kohn oos-**tehd keh ah**-bleh Een-**glehs?**
In case of emergency who do you want us to notify?	¿En caso de emergencia, a quién quiere que notifiquemos? Ehn kah-soh deh eh-mehr-**hen**-see-ah, ah kee-**ehn** kee-**eh**-reh **keh** noh-tee-fee-**keh**-mohs?
What type of insurance do you have?	¿Qué tipo de seguro tiene? **Keh** tee-poh deh seh-**goo**-roh **tee-eh**-neh?
__ None	__ Ninguno Neen-**goo**-noh

___ HMO / PPO

___ HMO / PPO
ah-che eh-meh oh / peh peh oh

___ Social security

___ Seguro social
Seh-**goo**-roh soh-see-ahl

___ Public aid

___ Ayuda pública
Ah-**yoo**-dah **poo**-blee-kah

Did you bring your insurance card?

¿Trajo su tarjeta de seguro?
Trah-hoh soo tahr-**heh**-tah deh seh-**goo**-roh?

What is his / her doctor's name?

¿Cuál es el nombre de su doctor?
Kwahl ehs ehl **nohm**-breh deh soo dohk-**tohr?**

What is your religion?

¿Cuál es su religión?
Kwahl ehs soo reh-lee-**hee-ohn?**

General Milestones

Etapas Generales

Eh-**tah**-pahs Heh-neh-**rah**-lehs

At what age did he / she start to:

A qué edad empezó a:
Ah **keh** eh-**dahd** ehm-peh-**soh** ah

___ smile

___ sonreir
sohn-reh-**eer**

___ sit up

___ sentarse
sehn-**tahr**-seh

___ roll over

___ voltearse
bohl-teh-**ahr**-seh

___ walk

___ caminar
kah-mee-**nahr**

___ say . . . mama, papa

___ decir . . . mamá, papá
deh-**seer** . . . mah-
mah, pah-**pah**

___ use two word sentences

___ usar oraciones con dos
palabras
oo-**sahr** oh-rah-**see-oh**-
nehs kohn dohs pah-**lah**-
brahs

Is he / she developing at the
same rate as siblings?

¿Se está desarrollando al
mismo paso que sus
hermanos?
Seh ehs-**tah** dehs-ah-rho-
yahn-doh ahl **mees**-moh pah-
soh **keh** soos ehr-**mah**-nohs?

Does he / she have any
problems with his / her
vision?

¿Tiene problemas con la vista?
Tee-eh-neh proh-**bleh**-mahs
kohn lah **bees**-tah?

Does he / she have any
problems hearing?

¿Tiene problemas al oir?
Tee-eh-neh proh-**bleh**-mahs
ahl oh-**eer?**

Do you have concerns about
your child's development?

¿Tiene preocupaciones acerca
del desarrollo de su niño (a)?
Tee-eh-neh preh-oh-koo-pah-
see-oh-nehs ah-**sehr**-kah dehl
dehs-ah-**rho**-yoh deh soo **nee**-
nyoh (ah)?

Milestones (by Age)

One Month

Can he / she lift the head while lying on his / her stomach?

Can he / she follow you with his / her eyes from one side to another?

Does he / she smile?

Does he / she smile when you play with him / her?

Two Months

Can he / she sustain his / her head steady while sitting up?

Etapas (por Edad)

Eh-**tah**-pahs pohr eh-**dahd**

Un Mes

Oon mehs

¿Puede él / ella levantar la cabeza mientras está acostado (a) boca abajo?
Pweh-deh ehl / eh-yah leh-bahn-**tahr** lah kah-**beh**-sah mee-**ehn**-trahs ehs-**tah** ah-kohs-**tah**-doh (ah) **boh**-kah ah-**bah**-hoh?

¿Puede él / ella seguirle a usted con sus ojos de un lado al otro?
Pweh-deh ehl / eh-yah seh-**geer**-leh ah oos-**tehd** kohn soos **oh**-hohs deh oon **lah**-doh ahl oh-troh?

¿Sonrie?
Sohn-**ree**-eh?

¿Sonrie cuando usted juega con él / ella?
Sohn-**ree**-eh **kwahn**-doh oos-**tehd** hoo-**eh**-gah kohn ehl / eh-yah?

Dos Meses

Dohs **meh**-sehs

¿Puede él / ella sostener su cabeza mientras está sentado (a)?
Pweh-deh ehl / eh-yah sohs-teh-**nehr** soo kah-**beh**-sah mee-**ehn**-trahs ehs-**tah** sehn-**tah**-doh (ah)?

Can he / she coo?	¿Puede él / ella hacer "agus"? Pweh-deh ehl / eh-yah ah-**sehr** ah-goos?
Does he / she laugh?	¿Él / ella se ríe? Ehl / eh-yah seh **ree**-eh?

Three Months

Tres Meses

Trehs **meh**-sehs

Can he / she support him / herself on legs with help?	¿Puede él / ella sostenerse en sus piernas con ayuda? Pweh-deh ehl / eh-yah sohs- teh-**nehr**-seh ehn soos **pee- ehr**-nahs kohn ah-**yoo**-dah?
Can he / she hold a toy?	¿Puede él / ella agarrar un juguete? Pweh-deh ehl / eh-yah ah-gah- **rhar** oon hoo-**geh**-teh?

Four Months

Cuatro Meses

Kwah-troh **meh**-sehs

Can he / she roll over in bed?	¿Puede él / ella voltearse en la cama? Pweh-deh ehl / eh-yah bohl- teh-**ahr**-seh ehn lah **kah**-mah?
Can he / she reach out toward objects?	¿Puede él / ella tender la mano hacia cosas? Pweh-deh ehl / eh-yah tehn- **dehr** lah **mah**-noh ah-see-ah koh-sahs?
Does he / she respond to voices of others?	¿Responde él / ella a voces de otros? Rehs-**pohn**-deh ehl / eh-yah ah **boh**-sehs deh oh-trohs?

Six Months

Seis Meses

Says **meh**-sehs

Does he / she sit without support?

¿Se sienta él / ella sin ayuda?
Seh see-**ehn**-tah ehl / eh-yah seen ah-**yoo**-dah?

Does he / she babble?

¿El / ella balbucea?
Ehl / eh-yah bahl-boo-**seh**-ah?

Seven to Nine Months

Siete a Nueve Meses

See-eh-teh ah **nweh**-beh **meh**-sehs

Can he / she stand holding onto things?

¿Puede él / ella pararse agarrándose de las cosas?
Pweh-deh ehl / eh-yah pah-**rahr**-seh ah-gah-**rhan**-doh-seh deh lahs **koh**-sahs?

Can he / she grasp with thumb and forefinger?

¿Puede él / ella agarrar con el pulgar y un dedo?
Pweh-deh ehl / eh-yah ah-gah-**rhar** kohn ehl pool-**gahr** ee con **deh**-doh?

Does he / she wave bye-bye?

¿Puede decir adiós con la mano?
Pweh-deh deh-**seer** ah-dee-**ohs** kohn lah **mah**-noh?

Does he / she point to things he / she wants?

¿Apunta a cosas que quiere?
Ah-**poon**-tah ah **koh**-sahs **keh** kee-**eh**-reh?

Eleven to Twelve Months

Once a Doce Meses

Ohn-seh ah **doh**-seh **meh**-sehs

Can he / she stand alone?

¿Puede él / ella pararse solo (la)?
Pweh-deh ehl / eh-yah pah-**rahr**-seh soh-loh (lah)?

Can he / she walk holding onto things?

¿Puede él / ella caminar agarrándose de las cosas?
Pweh-deh ehl / eh-yah kah-mee-**nahr** ah-gah-**rhan**-doh-seh deh lahs **koh**-sahs?

Does he / she say dada or mama?

¿Puede decir papá o mamá?
Pweh-deh deh-**seer** pah-**pah** oh mah-**mah?**

Thirteen to Fifteen Months

Trece a Quince Meses

Treh-seh ah **keen**-seh **meh**-sehs

Does he / she walk well?

¿Camina bien?
Kah-**mee**-nah bee-ehn?

Does he / she drink from a cup?

¿Toma de una taza?
Toh-mah deh **oo**-nah **tah**-sah?

Can he / she scribble?

¿Puede hacer garabatos?
Pweh-deh ah-**sehr** gah-rah-**bah**-tohs?

Can he / she say three to six words?

¿Puede decir de tres a seis palabras?
Pweh-deh deh-**seer** deh trehs a says pah-**lah**-brahs?

Does he / she imitate
activities?

¿Imita actividades?
Ee-**mee**-tah ahk-tee-bee-**dah**-
dehs?

Fifteen to Twenty Months

Quince a Veinte Meses

Keen-seh ah **beh-een**-teh
meh-sehs

Does the child run?

¿Corre el niño / la niña?
Koh-rhe ehl **nee**-nyoh / lah
nee-nyah?

Can he / she walk up steps?

¿Puede él / ella subir
escaleras?
Pweh-deh ehl / eh-yah soo-
beer ehs-kah-**leh**-rahs?

Can he / she feed him /
herself with a spoon?

¿Puede él / ella comer solo
(la) con una cuchara?
Pweh-deh ehl / eh-yah koh-
mehr soh-loh (lah) kohn **oo**-
nah koo-**chah**-rah?

Can he / she undress him /
herself?

¿Puede él / ella desvestirse
solo (la)?
Pweh-deh ehl / eh-yah dehs-
behs-**teer**-seh soh-loh (lah)?

Two to Two and a Half
Years

Dos a Dos Años y Medio

Dohs ah dohs **ah**-nyohs ee
meh-dee-oh

Can he / she kick a ball?

¿Puede él / ella patear una
pelota?
Pweh-deh ehl / eh-yah pah-
teh-**ahr oo**-nah peh **loh**-tah?

Can he / she walk up steps?

¿Puede él / ella subir
escaleras?
Pweh-deh ehl / eh-yah soo-
beer ehs-kah-**leh**-rahs?

Can he / she make a two-word phrase?

¿Puede él / ella hacer una frase de dos palabras?
Pweh-deh ehl / eh-yah ah-**sehr oo**-nah **frah**-seh deh dohs pah-**lah**-brahs?

Does he / she know six body parts?

¿Sabe él / ella seis partes del cuerpo?
Sah-beh ehl / eh-yah says **pahr**-tehs dehl **kwehr** poh?

Can he / she wash and dry his / her hands?

¿Puede él / ella lavarse y secarse las manos?
Pweh-deh ehl / eh-yah lah-**bahr** seh oo seh **kahr** seh lahs **mah**-nohs?

Can he / she put on any clothing?

¿Puede él / ella ponerse alguna ropa?
Pweh-deh ehl / eh-yah poh-**nehr**-seh ahl-**goo**-nah **roh**-pah?

Can he / she follow simple instructions?

¿Puede él / ella seguir instrucciones simples?
Pweh-deh ehl / eh-yah seh-**geer** eens-trook-**see-oh**-nehs **seem**-plehs?

Can he / she say his / her first and last names?

¿Puede él / ella decir su nombre y apellido?
Pweh-deh ehl / eh-yah deh-**seer** soo **nohm**-breh ee ah-peh-**yee**-doh?

Can he / she jump?

¿Puede él / ella saltar?
Pweh-deh ehl / eh-yah sahl-**tahr?**

Three to Four Years

Tres a Cuatro Años

Trehs ah **kwah**-troh **ah**-nyohs

Can he / she hop on one foot?

¿Puede él / ella brincar en un solo pie?
Pweh-deh ehl / eh-yah breen-**kahr** ehn oon soh-loh pee-eh?

Can he / she dress him / herself with supervision?

¿Puede él / ella vestirse con supervision?
Pweh-deh ehl / eh-yah behs-**teer**-seh kohn soo-pehr-bee-**see-ohn?**

Can he / she draw a figure with three parts?

¿Puede él / ella dibujar una figura con tres partes?
Pweh-deh ehl / eh-yah dee-boo-**har oo**-nah fee-**goo**-rah kohn trehs **pahr**-tehs?

Can he / she speak clearly?

¿Puede él / ella hablar claramente?
Pweh-deh ehl / eh-yah ah-**blahr** klah-rah-**mehn**-teh?

Does he / she know the name of a friend?

¿Él / ella sabe el nombre de un amigo?
Ehl / eh-yah sah-beh ehl **nohm**-breh deh oon ah-**mee**-goh?

Does he / she play in groups?

¿Él / ella juega en grupos?
Ehl / eh-yah hoo-**eh**-gah ehn **groo**-pohs?

Vaccines / Immunizations

Vacunas / Inmunizaciones

Bah-**koo**-nahs / een-moo-nee-
sah-**see-oh**-nehs

Do you have the child's
immunization record (card)
with you?

¿Trae con usted la tarjeta de
inmunización del niño (a)?
Trah-eh kohn oos-**tehd** lah
tahr-**he**-tah de een-moo-nee-
sah-**see-ohn** dehl **nee**-nyoh
(a)?

Is he / she up to date with the
vaccines?

¿Está al corriente con sus
vacunas?
Ehs-**tah** ahl koh-rhee-**ehn**-teh
kohn soos bah-**koo**-nahs?

How many vaccines has he /
she received?

¿Cuántas vacunas ha recibido
él / ella?
Kwahn-tahs bah-**koo**-nahs ah
reh-see-**bee**-doh ehl / eh-yah?

At what age did he / she
receive the last vaccine?

¿A qué edad recibió él / ella la
última vacuna?
Ah **keh** eh-dahd reh-see-bee-
oh ehl / eh-yah lah **ool**-tee-
mah bah-**koo**-nah?

___ Never

___ Nunca
Noon-kah

___ Two months

___ Dos meses
Dohs **meh**-sehs

___ Months ago

Hace ___ meses
Ah-seh   **meh**-sehs

When did he / she receive the last vaccine?

¿Cuándo recibió él / ella la última vacuna?
Kwahn-doh reh-see-bee-**oh** ehl / eh-yah lah **ool**-tee-mah bah-**koo**-nah?

Do you know which vaccines he / she received?

¿Sabe usted cuáles vacunas recibió?
Sah-beh oos-**tehd kwahl**-ehs bah-**koo**-nahs reh-see-bee-**oh?**

Do you know which vaccines he / she is missing?

¿Sabe usted cuáles vacunas le faltan?
Sah-beh oos-**tehd kwahl**-ehs bah-**koo**-nahs leh **fahl**-tahn?

Common Terms During the Exam for Vaccines

Your child is up to date with his / her vaccines.

Su niño / niña está al corriente con sus vacunas.
Soo **nee**-nyoh / **nee**-nyah ehs-**tah** ah koh-rhee-**ehn**-teh kohn soos bah-**koo**-nahs.

Your child is not up to date with his / her vaccines.

Su niño / niña no está al corriente con sus vacunas.
Soo **nee**-nyoh / **nee**-nyah noh ehs-**tah** ahl koh-rhee-**ehn**-teh kohn soos bah-**koo**-nahs.

Your child needs the vaccines today.

Su niño / niña necesita las vacunas hoy.
Soo **nee**-nyoh / **nee**-nyah neh-seh-**see**-tah lahs bah-**koo**-nahs oy.

Today, he / she can't receive the vaccines because he / she has . . .

Hoy, él / ella no puede recibir las vacunas porque tiene . . .
Oy, ehl / eh-yah noh pweh-deh reh-see-**beer** lahs bah-**koo**-nahs pohr-**keh tee-eh**-neh . . .

___ fever

___ fiebre
fee-eh-breh

cold

___ catarro / resfriádo
kah-**tah**-rho / rehs-free-**ah**-doh

___ ear infection

___ infección del oido
een-feg-**see-ohn** dehl oh-**ee**-doh

___ throat infection

___ infección de la garganta
een-feg-**see-ohn** deh lah gahr-**gahn**-tah

Your child needs the next vaccines in ___ months.

Su niño / niña necesita las próximas vacunas en ___ meses.
Soo **nee**-nyoh / **nee**-nyah neh-seh-**see**-tah lahs **prog**-see-mahs bah-**koo**-nahs ehn ___ meh-sehs.

Discharge Instructions for Vaccinations

Call your doctor or go to the hospital if he / she has . . .

Llame a su médico o vaya al hospital si él / ella tiene . . .
Yah-meh ah soo **meh**-dee-koh oh bah-yah ahl **ohs**-pee-tahl see ehl / eh-yah **tee-eh**-neh . . .

___ fever

___ fiebre
fee-eh-breh

___ vomiting

___ vómito
boh-mee-toh

___ seizures

___ convulsiones
kohn-bool-**see-ohn**-ehs

___ redness around the
injection

___ rojo alrededor de la
inyección
roh-ho ahl-rhe-deh-**dohr**
deh lah een-jeg-**see**-ohn

Return to the hospital if the
child is . . .

Regrese al hospital si el niño /
niña está . . .
Reh-**greh**-seh ahl **ohs**-pee-tahl
see ehl **nee**-nyoh / **nee**-nyah
ehs-**tah** . . .

___ crying a lot

___ llorando mucho
yoh-**rahn**-doh **moo**-choh

___ unconsolable

___ inconsolable
een-kohn-soh-**lah**-bleh

Bring the vaccination card
with you on the next visit.

Traiga la tarjeta de vacunación
con usted en la próxima visita.
Trah-ee-gah lah tahr-**he**-tah
deh bah-koo-nah-**see-ohn**
kohn oos-**tehd** ehn lah **prog**-
see-mah bee-**see**-tah.

Perinatal / Prenatal History

Historia Perinatal / Prenatal

Ees-**toh**-ree-ah peh-ree-nah-
tahl / preh-nah-**tahl**

How many children do you
have?

¿Cuántos niños tiene?
Kwahn-tohs **nee**-nyohs **tee-eh**-
neh?

How much did the child weigh at birth?

¿Cuánto pesó el niño al nacer?
Kwahn-toh peh-**soh** ehl **nee**-nyoh ahl nah-**sehr?**

How much does he / she weigh?

¿Cuánto pesa?
Kwahn-toh **peh**-sah?

___ pounds

___ libras
lee-brahs

___ kilograms

___ kilos
key-lohs

Was he / she born by vaginal delivery?

¿Nació por parto vaginal?
Nah-**see-oh** pohr **pahr**-toh bah-hee-**nahl?**

Was he / she born by C-section?

¿Nació por cesárea?
Nah-**see-oh** pohr seh-**sah**-reh-ah?

Did he / she have any breathing problems at birth?

¿Tuvo problemas de la respiración al nacer?
Too-boh proh-**bleh**-mahs deh lah rehs-pee-rah-**see-ohn** ahl nah-**sehr?**

Did he / she go home with you?

¿Se fué a casa con usted?
Seh **fweh** ah **kah**-sah kohn oos-**tehd?**

Was he / she hospitalized after birth?

¿Lo / la hospitalizaron después de nacer?
Loh / lah ohs-pee-tah-lee-**sah**-rohn dehs-**pwehs** deh nah-**sehr?**

How many days did he / she stay in the hospital?

¿Cuántos días se quedó en el hospital?
Kwahn-tohs **dee**-ahs seh keh-**doh** ehn ehl **ohs**-pee-tahl?

Did you have infections during the pregnancy?	¿Tuvo usted infecciones durante el embarazo? Too-boh oos-**tehd** een-feg-**see-oh**-nehs doo-rahn-teh ehl ehm-bah-**rah**-soh?
Did you smoke during the pregnancy?	¿Fumó usted durante el embarazo? Foo-**moh** oos-**tehd** doo-**rahn**-teh ehl ehm-bah-**rah**-soh?
Did you drink alcohol during the pregnancy?	¿Tomó usted alcohol durante el embarazo? Toh-**moh** oos-**tehd** ahl-**kohl** doo-**rahn**-teh ehl ehm-bah-**rah**-soh?
Did you take drugs during the pregnancy?	¿Usó drogas durante el embarazo? Oo-**soh droh**-gahs doo-**rahn**-teh ehl ehm-bah-**rah**-soh?
Did you receive prenatal care during the pregnancy?	¿Recibió cuidado prenatal durante el embarazo? Reh-see-bee-**oh** kwih-**dah**-doh preh-nah-**tahl** doo-**rahn**-teh ehl ehm-bah-**rah**-soh?

Key Words

At birth	Al nacer Ahl nah-**sehr**
Was born	Nació Nah-**see-oh**
The birth	Parto / nacimiento **Pahr**-toh / nah-see-mee-**ehn**-toh

Weight	Peso **Peh**-soh
Weighs: He, she, you (*unfamiliar*)	Pesa **Peh**-sah
Weighed: He, she, you (*unfamiliar*)	Pesó Peh-**soh**
The pregnancy	El embarazo Ehl ehm-bah-**rah**-soh

Pain

Dolor

Doh-**lohr**

Where does he / she have the pain?	¿Dónde tiene el dolor? **Dohn**-deh **tee-eh**-neh ehl doh-**lohr?**
When did the pain start?	¿Cuándo empezó el dolor? **Kwahn**-doh ehm-peh-**soh** ehl doh-**lohr?**
Where did the pain start?	¿Dónde empezó el dolor? **Dohn**-deh ehm-peh-**soh** ehl doh-**lohr?**
Does the pain go to another place?	¿Le va el dolor a otro lugar? Leh bah ehl doh-**lohr** ah oh-troh loo-**gahr?**
Point to where the pain goes.	Apunte a dónde le va el dolor. Ah-**poon**-teh ah **dohn**-deh leh bah ehl doh-**lohr.**

How long does the pain last?	¿Cuánto tiempo le dura el dolor? **Kwahn**-toh **tee-ehm**-poh leh **doo**-rah ehl doh-**lohr?**
___ seconds	___ segundos seh-**goon**-dohs
___ minutes	___ minutos mee-**noo**-tohs
___ hours	___ horas **oh**-rahs
___ constant	___ constante kohns-**tahn**-teh
Does the pain come and go?	¿Le va y viene el dolor? Leh bah ee bee-eh-neh ehl doh-**lohr**?
Is the pain constant?	¿Es el dolor constante? Ehs ehl doh-**lohr** kohns-**tahn**-teh?
What is the pain like?	¿Cómo es el dolor? **Koh**-moh ehs ehl doh-**lohr?**
___ Acute	___ Agudo Ah-**goo**-doh
___ Severe	___ Severo / fuerte Seh-**beh**-roh / **fwehr**-teh
___ Like a knife	___ Como cuchillo **Koh**-moh koo-**chee**-yoh
___ Soreness	___ Adolorido Ah-doh-loh-**ree**-doh
___ Burning	___ Quemante Keh-**mahn**-teh

___ Pressure

___ Like cramps

Has he / she had this type of
pain before?

___ Opresivo
Oh-preh-**see**-boh

___ Como calambres
Koh-moh kah-**lahm**-
brehs

¿Ha tenido él / ella este tipo
de dolor antes?
Ah teh-**nee**-doh ehl / eh-yah
ehs-teh tee-poh deh doh-**lohr**
ahn-tehs?

What things cause the pain?

___ Running

___ Walking

___ Bending

___ Breathing

___ Eating

___ Coughing

What makes the pain better?

___ Nothing

¿Qué cosas le causan el dolor?
Keh koh-sahs leh kah-oo-sahn
ehl doh **lohr?**

___ Correr
Koh-**rher**

___ Caminar
Kah-mee-**nahr**

___ Agacharse
Ah-gah-**char**-seh

___ Respirar
Rehs-pee-**rahr**

___ Comer
Koh-**mehr**

___ Toser
Toh-**sehr**

¿Qué le mejora el dolor?
Keh-leh meh-**hoh**-rah ehl doh-
lohr?

___ Nada
Nah-dah

___ Tylenol

___ Tylenol
Tay-leh-nohl

___ Sleeping

___ Dormir
Dohr-meehr

___ Eating

___ Comer
Koh-**mehr**

Does he / she have fever?

¿Tiene fiebre?
Tee-eh-neh **fee-eh**-breh?

Does he / she have vomiting?

¿Tiene vómito?
Tee-eh-neh **boh**-mee-toh?

Did he / she fall?

¿Se cayó?
Seh kah-**yoh?**

Did someone hit him / her?

¿Alguien le pegó?
Ahl-gee-ehn leh peh-**goh**?

Does he / she have trouble breathing?

¿Tiene problemas para respirar?
Tee-eh-neh proh-**bleh**-mahs pah-rah rehs-pee-**rahr?**

Is the pain

¿Es el dolor
Ehs ehl doh-**lohr**

___ the same

___ igual
ee-**gwahl**

___ better

___ mejor
meh-**hohr**

___ worse

___ peor
peh-**ohr**

since it started?

desde que empezó?
dehs-deh **keh** ehm-peh-**soh?**

Has he / she taken something for the pain?

¿Ha tomado algo para el dolor?
Ah toh-**mah**-doh ahl-goh pah-rah ehl doh-**lohr?**

___ Tylenol

___ Tylenol
Tay-leh-nohl

___ Aspirin

___ Aspirina
Ahs-pee-**ree**-nah

___ Ibuprofen

___ Ibuprofen
Ee-boo-proh-fehn

Common Terms During the Exam for Pain

Your child has . . .

Su niño / niña tiene . . .
Soo **nee**-nyoh / **nee**-nyah **tee-eh**-neh . . .

___ muscular pain

___ dolor muscular
doh-**lohr** moos-koo-**lahr**

___ colic

___ cólico
koh-lee-koh

___ fracture

___ fractura
frag-**too**-rah

___ sprain

___ torcedura
tohr-seh-**doo**-rah

___ infection

___ infección
een-feg-**see-ohn**

He / she needs an X-ray.

Él / ella necesita rayos equis.
Ehl / eh-yah neh-seh-**see**-tah-**rha**-yohs **eh**-keys.

He / she needs an ultrasound.

Él / ella necesita un ultrasonido.
Ehl / eh-yah neh-seh-**see**-tah
oon **ool**-trah-soh-**nee**-doh.

He / she needs pain medication.

Él / ella necesita medicina para el dolor.
Ehl / eh-yah neh-seh-**see**-tah
meh-dee-**see**-nah pah-rah ehl
doh-**lohr.**

He / she needs blood and urine tests.

Él / ella necesita pruebas de sangre y orina.
Ehl / eh-yah neh-seh-**see**-tah
proo-eh-bahs deh **sahn**-greh
ee oh-**ree**-nah.

Discharge Instructions for Pain

Give him / her Tylenol or Advil every __ hours for the pain.

Déle Tylenol o Advil cada __ horas para el dolor.
Dehl-leh Tay-leh-nohl oh Ad-
beel kah-dah __ **oh**-rahs
pah-rah ehl doh-**lohr.**

Return to the hospital if he / she has . . .

Regrese al hospital si él / ella tiene . . .
Reh-**greh**-seh ahl **ohs**-pee-tahl
see ehl / eh-yah **tee-eh**-
neh . . .

__ fever

__ fiebre
fee-eh-breh

__ vomiting

__ vómito
boh-mee-toh

Fever

Fiebre

Fee-eh-breh

When did the fever start?

¿Cuándo empezó la fiebre?
Kwahn-doh ehm-peh-**soh** lah
fee-eh-breh?

It has been ___ days

Hace ___ días
Ah-seh **dee**-ahs

___ today

___ hoy
oy

___ yesterday

___ ayer
ah-**yehr**

___ day before yesterday

___ ante ayer
ahn-teh ah-**yehr**

Does he / she have pain in the ears?

¿Tiene dolor en los oídos?
Tee-eh-neh doh-**lohr** ehn lohs
oh-**ee**-dohs?

Is he / she pulling at the ears?

¿Está jalándose / tirándose de
las orejas?
Ehs-**tah** hah-**lahn**-doh-seh /
tee-**rahn**-doh-seh deh lahs oh-
reh-has?

Is he / she drinking / eating well?

¿Está tomando / comiendo
bien?
Ehs-**tah** toh-**mahn**-doh / koh-
mee-**ehn**-doh bee-ehn?

Does he / she sleep more than usual?

¿Él / ella duerme más de lo
normal?
Ehl / eh-yah **dwehr**-meh mahs
deh loh nohr-**mahl?**

Does he / she cry more than usual?

¿Él / ella llora más de lo normal?
Ehl / eh-yah **yoh**-rah mahs deh loh nohr-**mahl?**

Do you have difficulty waking him / her up?

¿Tiene dificultad para despertarlo (la)?
Tee-eh-neh dee-fee-kool-**tahd** pah-rah dehs-pehr-**tahr**-loh (lah)?

Does he / she stop crying when you pick him / her up?

¿Deja de llorar cuando lo / la levanta?
Deh-hah deh yoh-**rahr kwahn**-doh loh / lah leh-**bahn**-tah?

Can you console him / her?

¿Puede consolarlo (la)?
Pweh-deh kohn-soh-**lahr**-loh (lah)?

Has he / she been active?

¿Ha estado activo (a)?
Ah ehs-**tah**-doh ahk-**tee**-boh (bah)?

Does he / she smile?

¿Él / ella sonrie?
Ehl / eh-yah sohn-**ree**-eh?

Does he / she play?

¿Él / ella juega?
Ehl / eh-yah **hweh**-gah?

Have you taken his / her temperature?

¿Le ha tomado la temperatura?
Leh ah toh-**mah**-doh lah tehm-peh-rah-**too**-rah?

How did you take his / her temperature?

¿Cómo le tomó la temperatura?
Koh-moh leh toh-**moh** lah tehm-peh-rah-**too**-rah?

___ By mouth

___ Rectally

___ Under his axilla

How high was his
temperature?

Have you given him / her
medicine for the fever?

___ Tylenol

___ Advil / Ibuprofen

When did you give him
medicine for the fever?

It has been ___ hours

___ days

___ Por la boca
Pohr lah **boh**-kah

___ Por el recto
Pohr ehl **reg**-toh

___ Debajo de la axila
Deh-bah-hoh deh lah ag-
see-lah

¿Cómo estaba de alta su
temperatura?
Koh-moh ehs-**tah**-bah deh
ahl-tah soo tehm-peh-rah-**too**-
rah?

¿Le ha dado medicina para la
fiebre?
Leh ah dah-doh meh-dee-**see**-
nah pah-rah lah **fee-eh**-breh?

___ Tylenol
Tay-leh-nohl

___ Advil / Ibuprofen
Ahd-beel / Ee-boo-proh-
fehn

¿Cuándo le dió medicina para
la fiebre?
Kwahn-doh leh dee-**oh** meh-
dee-**see**-nah pah-rah lah **fee-
eh**-breh?

Hace ___ horas
Ah-seh **oh**-rahs

___ días
dee-ahs

How much medicine did you give him / her?

¿Cuánta medicina le dió?
Kwahn-tah meh-dee-**see**-nah leh dee-**oh?**

___ Half a teaspoon

___ Media cucharada
Meh-dee-ah koo-chah-**rah**-dah

___ One teaspoon

___ Una cucharada
Oo-nah koo-chah-**rah**-dah

___ Two teaspoons

___ Dos cucharadas
Dohs koo-chah-**rah**-dahs

___ One dropper

___ Un gotero
Oon goh-**teh**-roh

___ Half a dropper

___ Medio gotero
Meh-dee-oh goh-**teh**-roh

Does he / she have chronic ear infections?

¿Tiene infecciones crónicas de los oídos?
Tee-eh-neh een-feg-**see-ohn**-ehs **kroh**-nee-kahs deh lohs oh-**ee**-dohs?

Does he / she complain of pain when he / she urinates?

¿Se queja de dolor cuando orina?
Seh **keh**-hah deh doh-**lohr kwahn**-doh oh-**ree**-nah?

Is he / she urinating more than normal?

¿Está orinando más de lo normal?
Ehs-**tah** oh-ree-**nahn**-doh mahs deh loh nohr-**mahl?**

Does he / she have a sore throat?

¿Tiene dolor de garganta?
Tee-eh-neh doh-**lohr** deh gahr-**gahn**-tah?

Is he / she drooling?

¿Está babeando?
Ehs-**tah** bah-beh-**ahn**-doh?

Does he / she have pain when swallowing food or saliva?

¿Tiene dolor para pasar la comida o la saliva?
Tee-eh-neh doh-**lohr** pah-rah pah-**sahr** lah koh-**mee**-dah oh lah sah-**lee**-bah?

Does he / she have a cough?

¿Tiene él / ella tos?
Tee-eh-neh ehl / eh-yah tohs?

Does he / she have phlegm?

¿Tiene flema?
Tee-eh-neh **fleh**-mah?

What color is it?

¿De qué color es?
Deh **keh** koh-**lohr** ehs?

___ White

___ Blanca
Blahn-kah

___ Yellow

___ Amarilla
Ah-mah-**ree**-yah

___ Green

___ Verde
Behr-deh

Does he / she have a runny nose?

¿Le está escurriendo a él / ella la nariz?
Leh ehs-**tah** ehs-koo-rhee-**ehn**-doh ah ehl / eh-yah lah nah-**rees?**

Does he / she have vomiting?

¿Tiene vómito?
Tee-eh-neh **boh**-mee-toh?

When was the last time he / she vomited?

¿Cuándo fué la última vez que vomitó?
Kwahn-doh **fweh** lah **ool**-tee-mah behs **keh** boh-mee-**toh?**

It has been ___ hours ___ days

Hace ___ horas ___ días
Ah-seh **oh**-rahs **dee**-ahs

How many times a day does he / she vomit?

¿Cuántas veces vomita al día?
Kwahn-tahs **beh**-sehs boh-**mee**-tah ahl **dee**-ah?

Have you noticed blood in the vomit?

¿Ha notado sangre en el vómito?
Ah noh-**tah**-doh **sahn**-greh ehn ehl **boh**-mee-toh?

Does he / she have diarrhea?

¿Tiene diarrea?
Tee-eh-neh dee-ah-**rhe-ah?**

How many times a day does he / she have diarrhea?

¿Cuántas veces al día tiene él / ella diarrea?
Kwahn-tahs **beh**-sehs ahl **dee**-ah **tee-eh**-neh ehl / eh-yah dee-ah-**rhe-ah?**

Have you noticed blood in the diarrhea?

¿Ha notado sangre en la diarrea?
Ah noh-**tah**-doh **sahn**-greh ehn lah dee-ah-**rhe-ah?**

Does he / she have pain in the abdomen?

¿Tiene dolor en el abdomen?
Tee-eh-neh doh-**lohr** ehn ehl ab-**doh**-mehn?

For how many days has he / she had pain in the abdomen?

¿Por cuántos días ha tenido dolor en el abdomen?
Pohr **kwahn**-tohs **dee**-ahs ah teh-**nee**-doh doh-**lohr** ehn ehl ab-**doh**-mehn?

Show me where the pain is.

Enséñeme dónde tiene el dolor.
Ehn-**seh**-nyeh-meh **dohn**-deh **tee-eh**-neh ehl doh-**lohr.**

Common Terms During the Exam for Fever

Your child has an ear
infection.

Su niño (a) tiene infección en
el oído.
Soo **nee**-nyoh (ah) **tee-eh**-neh
een-feg-**see-ohn** ehn ehl oh-
ee-doh.

Your child has a throat
infection.

Su niño (a) tiene infección en
la garganta.
Soo **nee**-nyoh (ah) **tee-eh**-neh
een-feg-**see-ohn** ehn lah gahr-
gahn-tah.

Your child has a viral
infection.

Su niño (a) tiene infección
viral.
Soo **nee**-nyoh (ah) **tee-eh**-neh
een-feg-**see-ohn** bee-**rahl.**

Your child has the flu.

Su niño (a) tiene gripa.
Soo **nee**-nyoh (ah) **tee-eh**-neh
gree-pah.

Your child has an infection in
the urine.

Su niño (a) tiene infección en
la orina.
Soo **nee**-nyoh (ah) **tee-eh**-neh
een-feg-**see-ohn** ehn lah-oh-
ree-nah.

Your child has pneumonia.

Su niño (a) tiene pulmonía.
Soo **nee**-nyoh (ah) **tee-eh**-neh
pool-moh-**nee**-ah.

Your child needs antibiotics.

Su niño (a) necesita
antibióticos.
Soo **nee**-nyoh (ah) neh-seh-
see-tah ahn-tee-bee-**oh**-tee-
kohs.

Your child needs intravenous antibiotics.

Su niño (a) necesita antibióticos intravenosos.
Soo **nee**-nyoh (ah) neh-seh-**see**-tah ahn-tee-bee-**oh**-tee-kohs een-trah-beh-**noh**-sohs.

We need to admit your child.

Necesitamos admitirlo (la) / internarlo (la).
Neh-seh-see-**tah**-mohs ahd-mee-**teer**-loh (lah) / een-tehr-**nahr**-loh (lah).

He / she needs to stay in the hospital for a few days.

El / ella necesita quedarse en el hospital por unos días.
Ehl / eh-yah neh-seh-**see**-tah keh-**dahr**-seh eh ehl **ohs**-pee-tahl pohr oo-nohs **dee**-ahs.

Discharge Instructions for Fever

Give him / her plenty of fluids.

Déle muchos líquidos.
Deh-leh **moo**-chohs lee-**kee**-dohs.

If he / she has a fever give him / her Tylenol every four hours for two days.

Si él / ella tiene fiebre déle Tylenol cada cuatro horas por dos días.
See ehl / eh-yah **tee-eh**-neh **fee-eh**-breh **deh**-leh tay-leh-nohl kah-dah **kwah**-troh **oh**-rahs pohr dohs **dee**-ahs.

Return to the hospital or see your doctor if the fever has not gone away in 2 days.

Regrese al hospital o vea a su médico si no se le quita la fiebre en 2 días.
Reh-**greh**-seh ahl **ohs**-pee-tahl oh beh-ah ah soo **meh**-dee-koh see noh seh leh kee-tah lah **fee-eh**-breh ehn dohs **dee**-ahs.

Return to the hospital if the child is not better or worse.

Regrese al hospital si el niño (a) no mejora o si se pone peor.
Reh-greh-seh ahl **ohs**-pee-tahl see ehl **nee**-nyoh (ah) noh meh-**hoh**-rah oh see seh poh-neh peh-**ohr.**

Return to the hospital if the child has . . .

Regrese al hospital si el niño / niña tiene . . .
Reh-**greh**-seh ahl **ohs**-pee-tahl see ehl **nee**-nyoh / **nee**-nyah **tee-eh**-neh . . .

___ convulsions

___ convulsiones
kohn-bool **see-oh** nohs

___ vomiting

___ vómito
boh-mee-toh

Neonatal Complaints

Fever (Neonatal)

Fiebre (Recién Nacido)

Fee-eh-breh (reh-see-**ehn** nah-**see**-doh)

When was the child born?

¿Cuándo nació el niño / la niña?
Kwahn-doh nah-**see-oh** ehl **nee**-nyoh / lah **nee**-nyah?

How old is he / she?

¿Cuánto tiene de edad?
Kwahn-toh **tee-eh**-neh deh eh-dahd?

___ days

___ días
dee-ahs

___ weeks

___ semanas
seh-**mah**-nahs

When did the fever start?

¿Cuándo empezó la fiebre?
Kwahn-doh ehm-peh-**soh** lah **fee-eh**-breh?

___ Today

___ Hoy
Oy

___ Yesterday

___ Ayer
Ah-**yehr**

It has been ___ days.

Hace ___ días.
Ah-seh ___ **dee**-ahs.

Did you take his / her temperature?

¿Le tomó la temperatura?
Leh toh-**moh** lah tehm-peh-rah-**too**-rah?

How did you take his / her temperature?

¿Cómo le tomó la temperatura?
Koh-moh leh toh-**moh** lah tehm-peh-rah-**too**-rah?

___ By mouth

___ Por la boca
Pohr lah **boh**-kah

___ Rectally

___ Por el recto
Pohr ehl **reg**-toh

___ Under his axilla

___ Debajo de la axila
Deh-**bah**-hoh deh lah ag-**see**-lah

How high was his / her temperature?

¿Cómo estaba de alta su temperatura?
Koh-moh ehs-**tah**-bah deh **ahl**-tah soo tehm-peh-rah-**too**-rah?

Have you given him / her medicine for the fever?

¿Le ha dado medicina para la fiebre?
Leh ah dah-doh meh-dee-**see**-nah pah-rah lah **fee-eh**-breh?

___ Tylenol

___ Tylenol
Tay-leh-nohl

___ Advil / Ibuprofen

___ Advil / Ibuprofen
Ahd-beel / Ee-boo-proh-fehn

When did you give him / her medicine for the fever?

¿Cuándo le dió medicina para la fiebre?
Kwahn-doh leh dee-**oh** meh-dee-**see**-nah pah-rah lah **fee-eh**-breh?

It has been ___ hours.

Hace ___ horas.
Ah-seh   **oh**-rahs

___ days

___ días
dee-ahs

How much medicine did you give him / her?

¿Cuánta medicina le dió?
Kwahn-tah meh-dee-**see**-nah leh dee-**oh?**

___ Half a teaspoon

___ Media cucharada
Meh-dee-ah koo-chah-**rah**-dah

___ One teaspoon

___ Una cucharada
Oo-nah koo-chah-**rah**-dah

___ Two teaspoons

___ Dos cucharadas
Dohs koo-chah-**rah**-dahs

___ One dropper

___ Un gotero
Oon goh-**teh**-roh

___ Half a dropper

___ Medio gotero
Meh-dee-oh goh-**teh**-roh

Does he / she have a cough?

¿Tiene tos?
Tee-eh-neh tohs?

Does he / she have vomiting?

¿Tiene vómito?
Tee-eh-neh **boh**-mee-toh?

Does he / she have diarrhea?

¿Tiene diarrea?
Tee-eh-neh dee-ah-**rhe-ah?**

Does he / she have difficulties breathing?

¿Tiene dificultades para respirar?
Tee-eh-neh dee-fee-kool-**tah**-dehs pah-rah rehs-pee-**rahr?**

Does he / she have nasal congestion or discharge?

¿Tiene congestión / deshecho de la nariz?
Tee-eh-neh kohn-hes-**tee-ohn** / des-**eh**-choh deh lah nah-**rees?**

Is his / her skin / eyes yellow in color?

¿Tiene la piel / los ojos de color amarillo?
Tee-eh-neh lah pee-**ehl** / lohs **oh**-hohs deh koh-**lohr** ah-mah-**ree**-yoh?

Is he / she taking the formula well?

¿Está tomando su fórmula bien?
Ehs-**tah** toh-**mahn**-doh soo **fohr**-moo-lah bee-ehn?

Is he / she crying more than usual?

¿Está llorando más de lo normal?
Ehs-**tah** yoh-**rahn**-doh mahs deh loh nohr-**mahl?**

Can you console him / her?

¿Lo / la puede consolar?
Loh / lah pweh-deh kohn-soh-**lahr?**

Does he / she stop crying when you hold him / her?

¿Deja de llorar cuando lo / la levanta?
Deh-hah deh yoh-**rahr kwahn**-doh loh / lah leh-**bahn**-tah?

Is he / she more irritable than usual?

¿Está más irritable de lo usual?
Ehs-**tah** mahs ee-ree-**tah**-bleh deh loh oo-soo-ahl?

Is he / she sleeping more than usual?

¿Está durmiendo más de lo usual?
Ehs-**tah** doohr-mee-**ehn**-doh mahs deh loh oo-soo-ahl?

Was he / she born by vaginal delivery?

¿Nació por parto vaginal?
Nah-**see-oh** pohr **pahr**-toh bah-hee-**nahl?**

Was he / she born by cesarean section?

¿Nació por cesárea?
Nah-**see-oh** pohr seh-**sah**-reh-ah?

Did you receive prenatal care during the pregnancy?

¿Recibió usted cuidado prenatal durante el embarazo?
Reh-see-**bee-oh** oos-**tehd** kwih-dah-doh preh-nah-**tahl** doo **rahn** teh ehl ehm-bah-**rah**-soh?

Did you have infections during the pregnancy?

¿Tuvo usted infecciones durante el embarazo?
Too-boh oos-**tehd** een-feg-**see-oh**-nehs doo-**rahn**-teh ehl ehm-bah-**rah**-soh?

___ Vaginal infection

___ Infección vaginal
Een-feg-**see-ohn** bah-hee-**nahl**

___ Urinary tract infection

___ Infección de la vía urinaria
Een-feg-**see-ohn** deh lah **bee**-ah oo-ree-**nah**-ree-ah

___ Skin infection

___ Infección de la piel
Een-feg-**see-ohn** deh lah pee-ehl

Did you receive antibiotics?

¿Recibió usted antibióticos?
Reh-see-**bee-oh** oos-**tehd** ahn-tee-bee-**oh**-tee-kohs?

Do you know if you had antibiotics at the time of delivery?

¿Sabe si le dieron a usted antibióticos al tiempo del parto?
Sah-beh see leh dee-**eh**-rohn ah oos-**tehd** ahn-tee-bee-**oh**-tee-kohs ahl **tee-ehm**-poh dehl **pahr**-toh?

Did the child receive antibiotics after birth?

¿Recibió antibióticos el niño / la niña después de nacer?
Reh-see-**bee-oh** ahn-tee-bee-**oh**-tee-kohs ehl **nee**-nyoh / lah **nee**-nyah dehs-**pwehs** deh nah-**sehr?**

Did the child go home with you after birth?

¿Se fué a casa con usted el niño / la niña después de nacer?
Seh **fweh** ah **kah**-sah kohn oos-**tehd** ehl **nee**-nyoh / lah **nee**-nyah dehs-**pwehs** deh nah-**sehr?**

How many days was he / she hospitalized?

¿Por cuántos días lo / la hospitalizaron?
Pohr **kwahn**-tohs **dee**-ahs loh / lah **ohs**-pee-tah-lee-**sah**-rohn?

Common Terms During the Exam for Fever (Neonatal)

We need to get a rectal temperature.

Necesitamos tomarle la temperatura por el recto.
Neh-seh-see-**tah**-mohs toh-**mahr**-leh lah tehm-peh-rah-**too**-rah pohr ehl **reg**-toh.

He / she needs blood and urine analysis.

Él / ella necesita análisis de sangre y orina.
Ehl / eh-yah neh-seh-**see**-tah ah-**nah**-lee-seehs deh **sahn**-greh ee oh-**ree**-nah.

He / she needs a chest X-ray.

Él / ella necesita una radiografía del pecho.
Ehl / eh-yah neh-seh-**see**-tah oo-nah **rah**-dee-oh-grah-**fee-ah** dehl **peh**-choh.

He / she needs intravenous fluid.

Él / ella necesita suero intravenoso.
Ehl / eh-yah neh-seh-**see**-tah soo-eh-roh een-trah-beh-**noh**-soh.

He / she needs intravenous antibiotics.

Él / ella necesita antibióticos intravenosos.
Ehl / eh-yah neh-seh-**see**-tah ahn too boo **oh** too kohs con trah-beh-**noh**-sohs.

I need to do a lumbar puncture.

Necesito hacerle una punción lumbar.
Noh sch **see** toh ah **sehr** lch oo-nah poon-**see-ohn** loom-**bahr.**

We need to know if he / she has meningitis.

Necesitamos saber si él / ella tiene meningitis.
Neh-seh-see-**tah**-mohs sah-**behr** see ehl / eh-yah **tee-eh**-neh meh-neen-**hee**-tees.

Meningitis is an infection of the brain.

Meningitis es una infección del cerebro.
Meh-neen-**hee**-tees ehs oo-nah een-feg-**see-ohn** dehl seh-**reh**-broh.

I am going to put a needle in his / her back to get spinal fluid.

Voy a ponerle una aguja en la espalda para sacarle líquido de la espina dorsal.
Boy ah poh-**nehr**-leh oo-nah ah-**goo**-hah ehn lah ehs-**pahl**-dah pah-rah sah-**kahr**-leh **lee**-kee-doh deh lah ehs-**pee**-nah dohr-**sahl.**

We must admit him / her.

Debemos admitirlo (la) / internarlo (la).
Deh-**beh**-mohs ad-mee-**teer**-loh (lah) / **een**-tehr-**nahr**-loh (lah).

Your child has an ear infection.

Su niño / niña tiene infección del oído.
Soo **nee**-nyoh / **nee**-nyah **tee-eh**-neh een-feg-**see-ohn** dehl oh-**ee**-doh.

Your child has an infection in the urine.

Su niño / niña tiene infección en la orina.
Soo **nee**-nyoh / **nee**-nyah **tee-eh**-neh een-feg-**see-ohn** ehn lah oh-**ree**-nah.

Your child has a viral infection.

Su niño / niña tiene infección viral.
Soo **nee**-nyoh / **nee**-nyah **tee-eh**-neh een-feg-**see-ohn** bee-**rahl**.

Your child has meningitis.

Su niño / niña tiene meningitis.
Soo **nee**-nyoh / **nee**-nyah **tee-eh**-neh meh-neen-**hee**-tees.

Apnea

Apnea

Ahp-neh-ah

What happened?

¿Que pasó?
Keh pah-**soh?**

Did he / she stop breathing?

¿Dejó de respirar?
Deh-**hoh** deh rehs-pee-**rahr?**

For how long did he / she stop breathing?

¿Por cuánto tiempo dejó de respirar?
Pohr **kwahn**-toh **tee-ehm**-poh deh-**hoh** deh rehs-pee-**rahr?**

___ seconds

___ segundos
seh-**goon**-dohs

___ minutes

___ minutos
mee-**noo**-tohs

Did he / she become blue?

¿Se puso morado (a)?
Seh poo-soh moh-**rah**-doh (dah)?

Did you find him / her face down?

¿Lo (la) encontró boca abajo?
Loh (lah) ehn-kohn-**troh boh**-kah ah-**bah**-hoh?

Did you find him / her face up?

¿Lo (la) encontró boca arriba?
Loh (lah) ehn-kohn-**troh boh**-kah ah-**rhee**-bah?

Was he / she stiff?

¿Estaba tieso (a)?
Ehs-**tah**-bah tee-**eh**-soh (ah)?

Was he / she floppy?

¿Estaba aguado (a)?
Ehs-**tah**-bah ah-goo-**ah**-doh?

Was he / she drooling?

¿Estaba babeando?
Ehs-**tah**-bah bah-beh-**ahn**-doh?

Did he / she start breathing on his / her own?

¿Empezó a respirar solo (sola)?
Ehm-peh-**soh** ah rehs-pee-**rahr** soh-loh (soh-lah)?

Did you give him / her mouth to mouth breathing?

¿Le dió respiración de boca a boca?
Leh dee-**oh** rehs-pee-rah-**see-ohn** deh **boh**-kah a **boh**-kah?

Did you notice vomit in his / her mouth?

¿Notó vómito en su boca?
Noh-**toh boh**-mee-toh ehn soo **boh**-kah?

Did you notice convulsions?

¿Notó convulsiones?
Noh-**toh** kohn-bool-**see-oh**-nehs?

Did he / she have a fever?

¿Tenía fiebre?
Teh-**nee**-ah **fee-eh**-breh?

Did he / she have a cold?

¿Tenía catarro?
Teh-**nee**-ah kah-**tah**-rho?

Was he / she acting normal today?

¿Estaba actuando normal hoy?
Ehs-tah-bah ahk-too-**ahn**-doh nohr-**mahl** oy?

Did he / she take his formula today?

¿Tomó su fórmula bien hoy?
Toh-**moh** soo **fohr**-moo-lah bee-ehn oy?

Did he / she have breathing problems before?

¿Tenía problemas de la respiración antes?
Teh-**nee**-ah proh-**bleh**-mahs deh lah rehs-pee-rah-**see-ohn ahn**-tehs?

Was he / she born premature?

¿Nació prematuro (a)?
Nah-**see-oh** preh-mah-**too**-roh (rah)?

Did he / she have breathing problems at birth?

¿Tuvo problemas de la respiración al nacer?
Too-boh proh-**bleh**-mahs deh lah rehs-pee-rah-**see-ohn** ahl nah-**sehr?**

Did he / she go home with you after the the the delivery?

¿Se fué a la casa con usted después de nacer?
Seh **fweh** ah lah **kah**-sah kohn oos-**tehd** dehs-**pwehs** deh nah-**sehr?**

How many days did he / she stay in the hospital?

¿Cuántos días se quedó en el hospital?
Kwahn-tohs **dee**-ahs seh keh-**doh** ehn ehl **ohs**-pee-tahl?

Common Terms for Apnea

Your child had a period of apnea.

Su niño (a) tuvo un ataque de apnea.
Soo **nee**-nyoh (ah) too-boh oon ah-**tah**-keh deh ap-neh-ah.

We have to admit him / her.

Necesitamos internarlo (la).
Neh-seh-see-**tah**-mohs **een**-tehr-**nahr**-loh (lah).

We need to put him / her on an apnea monitor.

Necesitamos ponerle un monitor de apnea.
Neh-seh-see-**tah**-mohs poh-**nehr**-leh oon moh-nee-**tohr** deh ap-neh-ah.

We need to observe his / her respirations.

Necesitamos observarle las respiraciones.
Neh-seh-see-**tah**-mohs ob-sehr-**bahr**-leh lahs rehs-pee-rah-**see-oh**-nehs.

He / she needs intravenous fluid.

Él / ella necesita suero / líquido intravenoso.
Ehl / eh-yah neh-seh-**see**-tah soo-eh-roh / **lee**-kee-doh een-trah-beh-**noh**-soh.

He / she needs oxygen.

Él / ella necesita oxígeno.
Ehl / eh-yah neh-seh-**see**-tah og-**see**-heh-noh.

Jaundice in the Newborn

Ictericia en el Recién Nacido

Eek-teh-**ree**-see-ah ehn ehl reh-**see-ehn** nah-**see**-doh

How old is he / she?

¿Cuánto tiene de edad?
Kwahn-toh **tee-eh**-neh deh eh-dahd?

___ days

___ días
dee-ahs

___ weeks

___ semanas
seh-**mah**-nahs

When did you notice that his / her skin is yellow?

¿Cuándo notó usted que su piel es amarilla?
Kwahn-doh noh-**toh** oos-**tehd keh** soo pee-ehl ehs ah-mah-**ree**-yah?

How many days after birth did his / her skin become yellow?

¿Cuántos días después de nacer se puso amarilla su piel?
Kwahn-tohs **dee**-ahs dehs-**pwehs** deh nah-sehr seh poo-soh ah-mah-**ree**-yah soo pee-ehl?

Did he / she have yellow skin / eyes when he / she was discharged from the hospital?

¿Tenía la piel / los ojos amarillos cuando le dieron de alta del hospital?
Teh-**nee**-ah lah pee-**ehl** / lohs **oh**-hohs ah-mah-**ree**-yohs **kwahn**-doh leh dee-**eh**-rohn deh **ahl**-tah dehl **ohs**-pee-tahl?

Do you breastfeed?

¿Le da pecho?
Leh dah **peh**-choh?

Do you give him / her formula?

¿Le da fórmula?
Leh dah **fohr**-moo-lah?

Does he / she have a fever?

¿Tiene fiebre?
Tee-eh-neh **fee-eh**-breh?

Does he / she have vomiting?

¿Tiene vómito?
Tee-eh-neh **boh**-mee-toh?

Is he / she feeding well?

¿Está comiendo bien?
Ehs-**tah** koh-mee-**ehn**-doh bee-ehn?

Is he / she irritable?

¿Está irritable?
Ehs-**tah** ee-ree-**tah**-bleh?

Can you console him / her?

¿Lo / la puede consolar?
Loh / lah pweh-deh kohn-soh-**lahr?**

Does he / she sleep well?

¿Duerme bien?
Dwehr-meh bee-ehn?

What color are his / her stools?

¿De qué color son sus excrementos?
Deh **keh** koh-**lohr** sohn soos egs-kreh-**mehn**-tohs?

___ Yellow

___ Amarillos
Ah-mah-**ree**-yohs

___ Green

___ Verdes
Behr-dehs

___ Clear

___ Claros
Klah-rohs

___ Black

___ Negros
Neh-grohs

Common Terms for Jaundice (Newborn)

I need to do blood tests.

Necesito hacerle pruebas de sangre.
Neh-seh-**see**-toh ah-**sehr**-leh **proo-eh**-bahs deh **sahn**-greh.

He / she has a high bilirubin level.

Él / ella tiene el nivel de la bilirubina alto.
Ehl / eh-yah **tee-eh**-neh ehl nee-**behl** deh lah bee-lee-roo-**bee**-nah **ahl**-toh.

He / she needs a lumbar puncture.

Él / ella necesita una punción lumbar.
Ehl / eh-yah neh-seh-**see**-tah oo-nah poon-**see-ohn** loom-**bahr.**

He / she has an infection.

Él / ella tiene una infección.
Ehl / eh-yah **tee-eh**-neh oo-nah een-feg-**see-ohn.**

He / she needs antibiotics.

Él / ella necesita antibióticos.
Ehl / eh-yah neh-seh-**see**-tah ahn-tee-bee-**oh**-tee-kohs.

He / she needs phototherapy.

Él / ella necesita fototerapia.
Ehl / eh-yah neh-seh-**see**-tah foh-toh-teh-**rah**-pee-ah.

We need to admit him / her.

Necesitamos internarlo (la).
Neh-seh-see-**tah**-mohs **een**-
tehr-**nahr**-loh (lah).

Discharge Instructions for Jaundice (Newborn)

Return to the hospital if he / she has . . .

Regrese al hospital si él / ella tiene . . .
Reh-**greh**-seh ahl **ohs**-pee-tahl
ooo ohl / oh yah **tee eh**-
neh . . .

___ fever

___ fiebre
fee-eh-breh

___ vomiting

___ vómito
boh-mee-toh

___ irritability

___ irritabilidad
ee-ree-tah-bee-lee-**dahd**

Pediatric Chief Complaints

PART **A**

Head and Neck

Earache

Dolor de Oído
Doh-**lohr** deh oh-**ee**-doh

For how many days has he / she had ear pain?

¿Por cuántos días ha tenido dolor de oído?
Pohr **kwahn**-tohs **dee**-ahs ah teh-**nee**-doh doh-**lohr** deh oh-**ee**-doh?

Which ear is he / she pulling?

¿Cuál oreja se está jalando?
Kwahl oh-**reh**-ha seh ehs-**tah** ha-**lahn**-doh?

___ Right

___ Derecha
Deh-**reh**-chah

___ Left

___ Izquierda
Ees-**kee-ehr**-dah

___ Both

___ Ambas
Ahm-bahs

Does he / she have a fever?

¿Tiene fiebre?
Tee-eh-neh **fee-eh**-breh?

For how many days has he / she had a fever?

¿Por cuántos días ha tenido fiebre?
Pohr **kwahn**-tohs **dee**-ahs ah teh-**nee**-doh **fee-eh**-breh?

Does he / she have vomiting?

¿Tiene vómito?
Tee-eh-neh **boh**-mee-toh?

Does he / she have diarrhea?

¿Tiene diarrea?
Tee-eh-neh dee-ah-**rhe-ah?**

Is he / she eating well?

¿Está comiendo bien?
Ehs-**tah** koh-mee-**ehn**-doh bee-ehn?

Is he / she taking his formula well?

¿Está tomando su fórmula bien?
Ehs-**tah** toh-**mahn**-doh soo **fohr**-moo-lah bee-ehn?

Is he / she crying more than normal?

¿Está llorando más de lo normal?
Ehs-**tah** yoh-**rahn**-doh mahs deh loh nohr-**mahl?**

Is he / she sleeping more than normal?

¿Está durmiendo más de lo normal?
Ehs-**tah** door-mee-**ehn**-doh mahs deh loh nohr-**mahl?**

Can you console the baby?

¿Puede consolar al bebé?
Pweh-deh kohn-soh-**lahr** ahl beh-**beh?**

Does he / she cry when you try to console him / her?

¿Llora cuando lo / la trata de consolar?
Yoh-rah **kwahn**-doh loh / lah trah-tah deh kohn-soh-**lahr?**

Is he / she acting normally?

¿Está actuando normal?
Ehs-**tah** ahk-too-**ahn**-doh nohr-**mahl?**

Has he / she had ear infections before?

¿Ha tenido infecciones de los oídos antes?
Ah teh-**nee**-doh een-feg-**see-oh**-nehs deh lohs oh-**ee**-dohs **ahn**-tehs?

Does he / she have abdominal pain?

¿Tiene dolor abdominal?
Tee-eh-neh doh-**lohr** ab-doh-mee-**nahl?**

Is he / she allergic to penicillin?

¿Es alérgico (a) a la penicilina?
Ehs ah-**lehr**-hee-koh (kah) ah lah peh-nee-see-**lee**-nah?

Common Terms for Earache

I am going to examine his / her ears.

Le voy a examinar los oídos.
Leh boy ah eg-sah-mee-**nahr** lohs oh-**ee**-dohs.

We need to take a rectal temperature.

Necesitamos tomarle la temperatura por el recto.
Neh-seh-see-**tah**-mohs toh-**mahr**-leh lah tehm-peh-rah-**too**-rah pohr ehl **reg**-toh.

Your child has an ear infection.

Su niño (a) tiene una infección en el oído.
Soo **nee**-nyoh (ah) **tee-eh**-neh **oo**-nah een-feg-**see-ohn** ehn ehl oh-**ee**-doh.

Your child needs antibiotics.

Su niño (a) necesita antibióticos.
Soo **nee**-nyoh (ah) neh-seh-**see**-tah ahn-tee-bee-**oh**-tee-kohs.

Your child has a lot of wax in his / her ears.

Su niño (a) tiene mucha cerilla en el oído.
Soo **nee**-nyoh (ah) **tee-eh**-neh **moo**-chah seh-**ree**-yah ehn ehl oh-**ee**-doh.

We need to clean the cerumen.

Necesitamos limpiar la cerilla.
Neh-seh-see-**tah**-mohs leem-pee-**ahr** lah seh-**ree**-yah.

Your child has a perforated eardrum.

Su niño (a) tiene la membrana del oído perforada.
Soo **nee**-nyoh (ah) **tee-eh**-neh lah mehm-**brah**-nah dehl oh-**ee**-doh pehr-foh-**rah**-dah.

Your child needs to see a specialist.

Su niño (a) necesita ver a un especialista.
Soo **nee**-nyoh (ah) neh-seh-**see**-tah behr ah oon ehs-**peh-see**-ah-lees-tah.

Discharge Instructions for Earache

Give him / her the antibiotic every ___ hours.

Déle el antibiótico cada ___ horas.
Deh-leh ehl ahn-tee-bee-**oh**-tee-koh kah-dah ___ **oh**-rahs.

Give him / her Tylenol every four hours if febrile.

Déle Tylenol cada cuatro horas si tiene fiebre.
Deh-leh ty-leh-nohl kah-dah **kwah**-troh **oh**-rahs see **tee-eh**-neh **fee-eh**-breh.

Give pediaprofen every six hours.

Déle pediaprofen cada seis horas.
Deh-leh peh-dee-ah-proh-fehn kah-dah says **oh**-rahs.

Return to the hospital if the child has . . .

Regrese al hospital si el niño (a) tiene . . .
Reh-**greh**-seh ahl **ohs**-pee-tahl see ehl **nee**-nyoh (ah) **tee-eh**-neh . . .

___ persistent fever

___ fiebre persistente
fee-eh-breh pehr-sees-**tehn**-teh

___ seizures / convulsions

___ ataques epilépticos / convulsiones
ah-**tah**-kehs eh-pee-**lep**-tee-kohs / kohn-bool-**see-oh**-nehs

___ vomiting

___ vómito
boh-mee-toh

See your doctor in ten days to recheck the ears or sooner if the child is not better.

Vea a su médico en diez días para revisarle los oídos o más pronto si no está mejor.
Beh-ah ah soo **meh**-dee-koh ehn dee-ehs **dee**-ahs pah-rah reh-bee-**sahr**-leh lohs oh-**ee**-dohs oh mahs **prohn**-toh see noh ehs-**tah** meh-**hor.**

Do not use Q-tips.

No use isopos.
Noh **oo**-seh ee-**soh**-pohs.

Sore Throat

Dolor de Garganta

Doh-**lohr** deh gahr-**gahn**-tah

For how many days has he / she had the pain?

¿Por cuántos días ha tenido él / ella el dolor?
Pohr **kwahn**-tohs **dee**-ahs ah teh-**nee**-doh ehl / eh-yah ehl doh-**lohr?**

Does he / she have pain upon swallowing?

¿Tiene él / ella dolor para pasar saliva?
Tee-eh-neh ehl / eh-yah doh-**lohr** pah-rah pah-**sahr** sah-**lee**-bah?

Can he / she drink fluids?

¿Puede él / ella tomar líquidos?
Pweh-deh ehl / eh-yah toh-**mahr lee**-kee-dohs?

Have you noticed a change in his / her voice?

¿Ha notado cambio en su voz?
Ah noh-**tah**-doh **kahm**-bee-oh ehn soo bohs?

Is he / she hoarse?

¿Está ronco (a)?
Ehs-**tah rohn**-koh (ah)?

Is he / she drooling?

¿Está babeando?
Ehs-**tah** bah-beh-**ahn**-doh?

Does he / she have a fever?

¿Tiene fiebre?
Tee-eh-neh **fee-eh**-breh?

Does he / she have trouble breathing?

¿Tiene problemas al respirar?
Tee-eh-neh proh-**bleh**-mahs ahl rehs-pee-**rahr?**

Does he / she have a cough?

¿Tiene tos?
Tee-eh-neh tohs?

Does he / she have an earache?

¿Tiene dolor de oído?
Tee-eh-neh doh-**lohr** deh oh-**ee**-doh?

Does he / she have a headache?

¿Tiene dolor de cabeza?
Tee-eh-neh doh-**lohr** deh kah-**beh**-sah?

Does he / she have abdominal pain?

¿Tiene dolor en el abdomen?
Tee-eh-neh doh-**lohr** ehn ehl ab-**doh**-mehn?

Does he / she have vomiting?

¿Tiene vómito?
Tee-eh-neh **boh**-mee-toh?

Has he / she had throat infections before?

¿Ha tenido infecciones en la garganta antes?
Ah teh-**nee**-doh een-feg-**see-ohn**-ehs ehn lah gahr-**gahn**-tah **ahn**-tehs?

Does he / she have a rash?

¿Tiene manchas / ronchas en
la piel?
Tee-eh-neh **mahn**-chahs /
rohn-chahs ehn lah pee-ehl?

Does he / she have allergies?

¿Tiene alergias?
Tee-eh-neh ah-**lehr**-hee-ahs?

Is he / she allergic to
penicillin?

¿Es alérgico (a) a la penicilina?
Ehs ah-**lehr**-hee-koh ah lah
peh-nee-see-lee-nah?

Common Terms During the Exam for Sore Throat

Open your mouth.

Abra la boca.
Ah-brah lah **boh**-kah.

Stick out your tongue.

Saque la lengua.
Sah-keh lah **lehn**-gwah.

Say AAH.

Diga AAH.
Dee-gah aaahhh.

I need to do a throat culture.

Necesito hacerle un cultivo de
garganta.
Neh-seh-**see**-toh ah-**sehr**-leh
oon kool-**tee**-boh deh gahr-
gahn-tah.

He / she has a throat
infection.

Él / ella tiene una infección
de la garganta.
Ehl / eh-yah **tee-eh**-neh **oo**-
nah een-feg-**see-ohn** deh lah
gahr-**gahn**-tah.

He / she has an abscess in the
tonsil.

Él / ella tiene un absceso en la
amígdala.
Ehl / eh-yah **tee-eh**-neh oon
ahb-**seh**-soh ehn lah ah-**meeg**-
dah-lah.

I am going to give him / her an injection.

Le voy a dar una inyección.
Leh boy ah dahr **oo**-nah een-jeg-**see-ohn.**

I am going to give him / her antibiotics for the infection.

Le voy a dar antibióticos para la infección.
Leh boy ah dahr ahn-tee-bee-**oh**-tee-kohs pah-rah lah een-feg-**see-ohn.**

Discharge Instructions for Sore Throat

See your doctor if . . .

Vea a su médico si . . .
Beh-ah ah soo **meh**-dee-koh see . . .

___ he / she has trouble breathing

___ tiene dificultad para respirar
tee-eh-neh dee-fee-kool-**tahd** pah-rah rehs-pee-**rahr**

___ he / she has trouble swallowing

___ tiene dificultad para tragar
tee-eh-neh dee-fee-kool-**tahd** pah-rah trah-**gahr**

___ the fever doesn't go away in 2 days

___ no se le quita la fiebre en dos días
noh seh leh kee-tah la **fee-eh**-breh ehn dohs **dee**-ahs

___ he / she is not feeling better

___ no se siente mejor
noh seh **see-ehn**-teh meh-**hor**

Give him Tylenol every ___ hours as needed for fever.

Déle Tylenol cada ___ horas si es necesario para la fiebre.
Deh-leh Tay-leh-nohl kah-dah ___ **oh**-rahs see ehs neh-seh-**sah**-ree-oh pah-rah lah **fee-eh**-breh.

Give him / her the antibiotic every ___ hours.

Déle el antibiótico cada ___ horas.
Deh-leh ehl ahn-tee-bee-oh-tee-koh kah-dah ___ **oh**-rahs.

Red Eye

Ojo Rojo

Oh-hoh **roh**-ho

How long has it been red?

¿Por cuánto tiempo lo tiene rojo?
Pohr **kwahn**-toh **tee-ehm**-poh loh **tee-eh**-neh **roh**-ho?

___ Today

___ Hoy
Oy

___ Days

___ Días
Dee-ahs

Was he / she hit in the eye?

¿Se pegó en el ojo?
Seh peh-**goh** ehn ehl **oh**-hoh?

Did he / she get dust in the eye?

¿Le entró polvo en el ojo?
Leh ehn-**troh pohl**-boh ehn ehl **oh**-hoh?

Did he / she splash something in his / her eye?

¿Se salpicó con algo en el ojo?
Seh sahl-pee-**koh** kohn ahl-goh ehn ehl **oh**-hoh?

Did anyone stick a finger in his / her eye?

¿Alguien le picó el ojo con un dedo?
Ahl-gee-ehn leh pee-**koh** ehl **oh**-hoh kohn oon **deh**-doh?

Does he / she have eye discharge?

¿Tiene deshecho del ojo?
Tee-eh-neh dehs-**eh**-choh dehl **oh**-hoh?

What color is it?

¿De qué color es?
Deh **keh** koh-**lohr** ehs?

___ Clear

___ Claro
Klah-roh

___ Yellow

___ Amarillo
Ah-mah-**ree**-yho

___ Green

___ Verde
Behr-deh

Does he / she complain of pain in the eye?

¿Se queja de dolor en el ojo?
Seh **keh**-hah deh doh-**lohr** ehn ehl **oh**-hoh?

Does he / she wake up in the morning with his eyes glued shut?

¿Se levanta en la mañana con los ojos cerrados por el deshecho?
Seh leh-**bahn**-tah ehn lah mah-**nyah**-nah kohn lohs **oh**-hohs seh-**rha**-dohs pohr ehl dehs-**eh**-choh?

Do his / her eyes tear?

¿Le lloran los ojos?
Leh **yoh**-rahn lohs **oh**-hohs?

Does he / she complain of itching in the eyes?

¿Se queja de comezón en los ojos?
Seh **keh**-hah deh koh-meh-**sohn** ehn lohs **oh**-hohs?

Does he / she complain of burning in the eyes?

¿Se queja de ardor en los ojos?
Seh **keh**-hah deh ahr-**dohr** ehn lohs **oh**-hohs?

Does the light bother his / her eyes?

¿Le molesta la luz a sus ojos?
Leh moh-**lehs**-tah lah loos ah soos **oh**-hohs?

Did you put medicine in his / her eye?

¿Le puso medicina en el ojo?
Leh poo-soh meh-dee-**see**-nah ehn ehl **oh**-hoh?

Did you put eye drops?

¿Le puso gotas para los ojos?
Leh poo-soh **goh**-tahs pah-rah lohs **oh**-hohs?

Did you put eye ointment?

¿Le puso pomada para los ojos?
Leh poo-soh poh-**mah**-dah pah-rah lohs **oh**-hohs?

Common Terms During the Exam for Red Eye

Look at the light.

Mire la luz.
Mee-reh lah loos.

I am going to give him / her anesthetic eye drops.

Voy a darle gotas con anestesia.
Boy ah **dahr**-leh **goh**-tahs kohn ah-nehs-**teh**-see-ah.

Your child has a viral infection.

Su niño (a) tiene una infección viral.
Soo **nee**-nyoh (ah) **tee-eh**-neh oo-nah een-feg-**see-ohn** bee-**rahl**.

Your child has a bacterial infection.

Su niño (a) tiene una infección bacterial.
Soo **nee**-nyoh (ah) **tee-eh**-neh oo-nah een-feg-**see-ohn** bahk-teh-ree-**ahl.**

Your child has a corneal abrasion.

Su niño (a) tiene una raspadura (rasguño) en la cornea.
Soo **nee**-nyoh (ah) **tee-eh**-neh oo-nah rahs-pah-**doo**-rah (rahs-**goo**-nyoh) ehn lah **kohr**-neh-ah.

We are going to put ointment in his / her eye and patch it.

Vamos a ponerle pomada en el ojo y cubrirle el ojo con un parche.
Bah-mohs ah poh-**nehr**-leh poh-**mah**-dah ehn ehl **oh**-hoh ee koo-**breer**-leh ehl **oh**-hoh kohn oon **pahr**-cheh.

Discharge Instructions for Red Eye

Return to the hospital if he / she is not better in 2 days.

Regrese al hospital si no está mejor en dos días.
Reh-**greh**-seh ahl **ohs**-pee-tahl see noh ehs-**tah** meh-**hohr** ehn dohs **dee**-ahs.

Come back sooner if worse.

Regrese antes si está peor.
Reh-**greh**-seh ahn-tehs see ehs-**tah** peh-**ohr.**

Wash your hands after applying the medicine.

Lávese las manos después de ponerle la medicina.
Lah-beh-seh lahs **mah**-nohs dehs-**pwehs** deh poh-**nehr**-leh lah meh-dee-**see**-nah.

Use the medication ___ drops ___ times a day.

Use la medicina ___ gotas ___ veces al día.
Oo-seh lah meh-dee-**see**-nah ___ **goh**-tahs ___ **beh**-sehs ahl **dee**-ah.

See your doctor on _____.

Vea a su médico el _____.
Beh-ah ah soo **meh**-dee-koh ehl _____.

Don't remove his / her patch until you see the eye specialist.

No le quite el parche hasta que lo / la vea el especialista de los ojos.
Noh leh kee-teh ehl **pahr**-cheh ahs-tah **keh** lob / lah beah ehl ehs-**peh-see**-ah-lees-tah deh lohs **oh**-hohs.

Neck Mass

Bola en el Cuello

Boh-lah ehn ehl **kweh**-yoh

How long has there been neck swelling?

¿Cuánto tiempo lleva con la hinchazón en el cuello?
Kwahn-toh **tee-ehm**-poh **yeh**-bah kohn lah een-chah-**sohn** ehn ehl **kweh**-yoh?

It's been ___ hours ___ days.

Hace ___ horas ___ días.
Ah-seh ___ **oh**-rahs ___ **dee**-ahs.

Does he / she have problems swallowing?

¿Tiene problemas al tragar?
Tee-eh-neh proh-**bleh**-mahs ahl trah-**gahr?**

Does he / she have problems breathing?

¿Tiene problemas al respirar?
Tee-eh-neh proh-**bleh**-mahs ahl rehs-pee-**rahr?**

Does he / she have fever?

¿Tiene fiebre?
Tee-eh-neh **fee-eh**-breh?

Does he /she have pain in the neck?

¿Tiene dolor en el cuello?
Tee-eh-neh doh-**lohr** ehn ehl **kweh**-yoh?

Does he / she have pain in the ears?

¿Tiene dolor en los oídos?
Tee-eh-neh doh-**lohr** ehn lohs oh-**ee**-dohs?

Does he / she have pain in the teeth?

¿Tiene dolor en los dientes?
Tee-eh-neh doh-**lohr** ehn lohs dee-**ehn**-tehs?

Does he / she have sore throat?

¿Tiene dolor de garganta?
Tee-eh-neh doh-**lohr** deh gahr-**gahn**-tah?

Has he / she had the flu or a cold?

¿Ha tenido la gripa o catarro?
Ah teh-**nee**-doh lah **gree**-pah oh kah-**tah**-rho?

Is the mass getting bigger?

¿Le ha estado creciendo la bola?
Leh ah ehs-**tah**-doh kreh-see-**ehn**-doh lah boh-lah?

Does the mass move?

¿Se le mueve la bola?
Seh leh **mweh**-beh lah boh-lah?

Is the mass hard?

¿Es la bola de consistencia dura?
Ehs lah boh-lah deh kohn-sees-**tehn**-see-ah **doo**-rah?

Is the mass soft?

¿Es la bola de consistencia suave?
Ehs lah boh-lah deh kohn-sees-**tehn**-see-ah soo-**ah**-beh?

Has he / she lost weight?	¿Ha perdido peso? Ah pehr-**dee**-doh **peh**-soh?
Does he / she have night sweats?	¿Tiene sudores en la noche? **Tee-eh**-neh soo-**doh**-rehs ehn lah **noh**-cheh?
Has he / she been exposed to tuberculosis?	¿Ha sido expuesto a la tuberculosis? Ah see-doh eqs-**pwehs**-toh ah lah too-**behr**-koo-**loh**-sees?

Common Terms for Neck Mass

I need to take an X-ray.	Necesito sacarle una radiografía. Neh-seh-**see**-toh sah-**kahr**-leh **oo**-nah **rah**-dee-oh-grah-**fee-ah.**
I need to do a blood test.	Necesito hacerle una prueba de sangre. Neh-seh-**see**-toh ah-**sehr**-leh **oo**-nah **proo-eh**-bah deh **sahn**-greh.
Your child has an infection in . . .	Su niño (a) tiene una infección en . . . Soo **nee**-nyoh (ah) **tee-eh**-neh **oo**-nah een-feg-**see-ohn** ehn . . .
___ the throat	___ la garganta lah gahr-**gahn**-tah
___ the ears	___ los oídos lohs oh-**ee**-dohs

Your child has tooth abscess.

Su niño (a) tiene un absceso en el diente.
Soo **nee**-nyoh (ah) **tee-eh**-neh oon ab-**seh**-soh ehn ehl dee-**ehn**-teh.

I need to do a needle aspiration of the mass.

Necesito aspirarle la bola con una aguja.
Neh-seh-**see**-toh ahs-pee-**rahr**-leh lah boh-lah kohn oo-nah ah-**goo**-hah.

I need to drain the mass.

Necesito vaciarle la bola.
Neh-seh-**see**-toh bah-see-**ahr**-leh lah boh-lah.

Discharge Instructions for Neck Mass

Give him / her medicine ___ times a day.

Déle la medicina ___ veces al día.
Deh-leh lah meh-dee-**see**-nah ___ **beh**-sehs ahl **dee**-ah.

Give him / her Tylenol ___ times a day.

Déle Tylenol ___ veces al día.
Deh-leh **tay**-leh-nohl ___ **beh**-sehs ahl **dee**-ah.

Return to the hospital if . . .

Regrese al hospital si . . .
Reh-**greh**-seh ahl **ohs**-pee-tahl see . . .

___ he / she has a fever

___ él / ella tiene fiebre
ehl / eh-yah **tee-eh**-neh **fee-eh**-breh

___ the neck mass gets
bigger

___ la bola en el cuello crece
más
lah boh-lah ehn ehl
kweh-yoh **kreh**-seh
mahs

___ he / she has vomiting

___ él / ella tiene vómito
ehl / eh-yah **tee-eh**-neh
boh-mee-toh

___ he / she has difficulty
breathing

él / ella tiene dificultad
para respirar
ehl / eh-yah **tee-eh**-neh
dee-fee-kool-**tahd** pah-
rah rehs-pee-**rahr**

Cardiovascular
Respiratory

Shortness of Breath and Asthma

Falta de Aire y Asma

Fahl-tah deh ay-reh ee **ahs**-mah

For how many days has he / she had trouble breathing?

¿Por cuántos días ha tenido dificultad para respirar?
Pohr **kwahn**-tohs **dee**-ahs ah teh-**nee**-doh dee-fee-kool-**tahd** pah-rah rehs-pee-**rahr?**

Does he / she have a cough?

¿Tiene tos?
Tee-eh-neh tohs?

When did the cough start?

¿Cuándo empezó la tos?
Kwahn-doh ehm-peh-**soh** lah tohs?

It has been ___ hours.

Hace ___ horas.
ah-seh   **oh**-rahs

___ days

___ días
dee-ahs

___ weeks

___ semanas
seh-**mah**-nahs

Does he / she have phlegm with the cough?

¿Tiene flema con la tos?
Tee-eh-neh **fleh**-mah kohn lah tohs?

What color is it?

¿De qué color es?
Deh **keh** koh-**lohr** ehs?

___ White

___ Blanca
Blahn-kah

___ Yellow

___ Amarilla
Ah-mah-**ree**-yah

___ Green

___ Verde
Behr-deh

Do you believe the baby aspirated something (toy or peanut)?

¿Usted cree que el bebé aspiró algo (juguete o cacahuate)?
Oos-**tehd** kreh-eh keh ehl beh-**beh** ahs-pee-**roh** ahl-goh (hoo-**geh**-teh oh kah-kah-**hwah**-teh)?

Does he / she have fever?

¿Tiene fiebre?
Tee-eh-neh **fee-eh**-breh?

For how many ___ days ___ hours?

¿Por cuántos ___ días ___ horas?
Pohr **kwahn**-tohs ___ **dee**-ahs ___ **oh**-rahs?

Does he / she have asthma?

¿Tiene asma?
Tee-eh-neh **ahs**-mah?

What medicine does he / she take for asthma?

¿Qué medicina toma para el asma?
Keh meh-dee-**see**-nah **toh**-mah pah-rah ehl **ahs**-mah?

___ Ventolin

___ Ventolina
Behn-toh-lee-nah

___ Theodur

___ Theodur
Teoh-duhr

___ Prednisone

___ Prednisona
Prehd-nee-soh-nah

___ Azmacort

___ Azmacort
Ahs-mah-kohrt

How many times a day does
he / she take the medicine?

¿Cuántas veces al día toma la
medicina?
Kwahn-tahs **beh**-sehs ahl **dee**-
ah **toh**-mah lah meh-dee-**see**-
nah?

When was the last time he /
she took the medicine?

¿Cuándo fué la última vez que
tomó la medicina?
Kwahn-doh **fweh** lah ool-tee-
mah behs keh toh-**moh** lah
meh-dee-**see**-hah?

___ hours ___ days

___ horas ___ días
oh-rahs   **dee**-ahs

Is this attack similar to his /
her usual attacks?

¿Es este ataque similar a sus
ataques anteriores?
Ehs ehs-teh ah-**tah**-keh see-
mee-**lahr** ah soos ah-**tah**-kehs
ahn-teh-ree-**oh**-rehs?

Is this attack worse than other
attacks?

¿Es este ataque peor que
ataques anteriores?
Ehs ehs-teh ah-**tah**-keh peh-
ohr keh ah-**tah**-kehs ahn-teh-
ree-**oh**-rehs?

Do you give him / her
nebulized treatments at home?

¿Le da tratamientos de
nebulización en casa?
Leh dah trah-tah-mee-**ehn**-tohs
deh neh-boo-lee-sah-**see-ohn**
ehn **kah**-sah?

How many treatments did you
give him / her today?

¿Cuántos tratamientos le dió
hoy?
Kwahn-tohs trah-tah-mee-**ehn**-
tohs leh dee-**oh** oy?

When did you give him / her
the last treatment?

¿Cuándo le dió el último
tratamiento?
Kwahn-doh leh dee-**oh** ehl
ool-tee-moh trah-tah-mee-**ehn**-
toh?

Is he / she taking prednisone
now?

¿Está tomando prednisona
ahora?
Ehs-**tah** toh-**mahn**-doh prehd-
nee-soh-nah ah-oh-rah?

When did he / she take
prednisone last?

¿Cuándo fué la última vez que
tomó prednisona?
Kwahn-doh **fweh** lah **ool**-tee-
mah behs keh toh-**moh** prehd-
nee-soh-nah?

—— Today

—— Hoy
Oy

—— Yesterday

—— Ayer
Ah-**yehr**

—— Last week

—— La semana pasada
Lah seh-**mah**-nah pah-
sah-dah

—— Few weeks ago

—— Hace pocas semanas
Ah-seh poh-kahs seh-
mah-nahs

—— Cannot remember

—— No se acuerda
Noh seh ah-**kwehr**-dah

Do you believe that his / her
condition worsened because
of . . .

Usted cree que su condición
empeoró por . . .
Oos-**tehd** kreh-eh **keh** soo
kohn-dee-**see-ohn** ehm-peh-
oh-**roh** pohr . . .

___ change in the environment / weather

___ cambio del ambiente / clima
kahm-bee-oh dehl ahm-bee-**ehn**-teh / **klee**-mah

___ dust

___ polvo
pohl-boh

___ cigarette smoke

___ humo de cigarillo
oo-moh deh see-gah-**ree**-yoh

___ after running / exercise

___ después de correr / hacer ejercicio
dehs-**pwehs** deh koh-**rhehr** / ah-**sehr** eh-her-**see**-see-oh

How many times has he / she been hospitalized for asthma attacks this year?

¿Cuántas veces ha sido hospitalizado por ataques de asma este año?
Kwahn-tahs **beh**-sehs ah see-doh ohs-pee-tah-lee-**sah**-doh pohr ah-**tah**-kehs deh **ahs**-mah ehs-teh **ah**-nyoh?

How many times did he / she go to the emergency room for asthma attacks this year?

¿Cuántas veces ha ido a la sala de emergencia por ataques de asma este año?
Kwahn-tahs **beh**-sehs ah ee-doh ah lah sah-lah deh eh-mehr-**hen**-see-ah pohr ah-**tah**-kehs deh **ahs**-mah ehs-teh **ah**-nyoh?

How many times has he / she been hospitalized in intensive care for asthma?

¿Cuántas veces ha sido hospitalizado por ataques de asma en cuidado intensivo?
Kwahn-tahs **beh**-sehs ah see-doh ohs-pee-tah-lee-**sah**-doh pohr ah-**tah**-kehs deh **ahs**-mah ehn kwih-**dah**-doh een-tehn-**see**-boh?

Has he / she ever been intubated?

¿Alguna vez lo / la han intubado?
Ahl-**goo**-nah behs loh / lah ahn een-too-**bah**-doh?

Does his / her chest wheeze or have a whistling sound?

¿Le chifla el pecho o tiene silbido?
Leh **chee**-flah ehl **peh**-choh oh **tee-eh**-neh seel-**bee**-doh?

Do you have curtains in the child's room?

¿Tiene cortinas en el cuarto del niño (a)?
Tee-eh-neh kohr-**tee**-nahs ehn ehl **kwahr**-toh dehl **nee**-nyoh (ah)?

Do you have carpeting in the child's room?

¿Tiene alfombra en el cuarto del niño (a)?
Tee-eh-neh ahl-**fohm**-brah ehn ehl **kwahr**-toh dehl **nee**-nyoh (ah)?

Do you have stuffed animals in the child's room?

¿Tiene animales de peluche en el cuarto del niño (a)?
Tee-eh-neh ah-nee-**mah**-lehs deh peh-**loo**-cheh ehn ehl **kwahr**-toh dehl **nee**-nyoh (ah)?

Is there someone who smokes in the house?

¿Hay alguien que fume en la casa?
Ay **ahl**-gee-ehn **keh** foo-meh ehn lah **kah**-sah?

Do you have animals (cat, dog) in the house?

¿Tiene animales (gato, perro) en la casa?
Tee-eh-neh ah-nee-**mah**-lehs (gah-toh, peh-rho) ehn lah **kah**-sah?

Do you have cockroaches in the house?

¿Tiene cucarachas en la casa?
Tee-eh-neh koo-kah-**rah**-chahs ehn lah **kah**-sah?

Common Terms During the Exam for Shortness of Breath and Asthma

We need to do an X-ray of the chest.

Necesitamos hacerle una radiografía del pecho.
Neh-seh-see-**tah**-mohs ah-**sehr**-leh **oo**-nah **rah**-dee-oh-grah-**fee-ah** dehl **peh**-choh.

Your child needs a nebulized treatment.

Su niño (a) necesita un tratamiento de nebulización.
Soo **nee**-nyoh (ah) neh-seh-**see**-tah oon trah-tah-mee-**ehn**-toh deh neh-boo-lee-sah-**see-ohn.**

Your child needs an IV.

Su niño (a) necesita suero intravenoso.
Soo **nee**-nyoh (ah) neh-seh-**see**-tah soo-eh-roh een-trah-beh-**noh**-soh.

Your child has pneumonia.

Su niño (a) tiene pulmonía.
Soo **nee**-nyoh (ah) **tee-eh**-neh pool-moh-**nee-ah.**

Your child has asthma.

Su niño (a) tiene asma.
Soo **nee**-nyoh (ah) **tee-eh**-neh
ahs-mah.

Your child has the flu.

Su niño (a) tiene gripa.
Soo **nee**-nyoh (ah) **tee-eh**-neh
gree-pah.

We need to admit the child.

Necesitamos internar al
niño (a).
Neh-seh-see-**tah**-mohs een-
tehr-**nahr** ahl **nee**-nyoh (ah).

Your child needs more
treatments.

Su niño (a) necesita más
tratamientos.
Soo **nee**-nyoh (ah) neh-seh-
see-tah mahs trah-tah-mee-
ehn-tohs.

Your child needs oxygen.

Su niño (a) necesita oxígeno.
Soo **nee**-nyoh(ah) neh-seh-
see-tah og-**see**-heh-noh.

I need to do an arterial blood
gas.

Necesito hacerle un examen
de sangre arterial.
Neh-seh-see-toh ah-**sehr**-leh
oon eg-**sah**-mehn deh **sahn**-
greh ahr-teh-ree-**ahl.**

I need to know if your child
needs oxygen.

Necesito saber si su niño (a)
necesita oxígeno.
Neh-seh-see-toh sah-**behr** see
soo **nee**-nyoh (ah) neh-seh-
see-tah og-**see**-heh-noh.

Discharge Instructions for Shortness of Breath and Asthma

1. Return to the hospital if he / she is still short of breath or is not getting better.

1. Regrese al hospital si sigue con falta de aire o si no mejora.
Reh-**greh**-seh ahl **ohs**-pee-tahl see see-geh kohn fahl-tah deh ay-reh oh see noh meh-**ho**-rah.

2. Give him / her the medications as indicated.

2. Déle las medicinas como le indicaron.
Deh-leh lahs meh-dee-**see**-nahs **koh**-moh leh een-dee-**kah**-rohn.

3. Return to the hospital if . . .

3. Regrese al hospital si . . .
Reh-**greh**-seh ahl **ohs**-pee-tahl see . . .

___ the child has a fever

___ el niño / la niña tiene fiebre
ehl **nee**-nyoh / lah **nee**-nyah **tee-eh**-neh **fee-eh**-breh

___ has more shortness of breath

___ tiene más falta de aire
tee-eh-neh mahs fahl-tah deh ay-reh

___ the child has vomiting

___ el niño / la niña tiene vómito
ehl **nee**-nyoh / lah **nee**-nyah **tee-eh**-neh **boh**-mee-toh

Key Words / Phrases for Shortness of Breath and Asthma

To breathe (verb)	**Respirar** Rehs-pee-**rahr**
To aspirate (verb)	**Aspirar** Ahs-pee-**rahr**
To cough (verb)	**Toser** Toh-**sehr**
Aspirated (past tense)	**Aspiró** Ahs-pee-**roh**
The cough (noun)	**La tos** Lah tohs
Attack (noun)	**Ataque** Ah-**tah**-keh
Treatment	**Tratamiento** Trah-tah-mee-**ehn**-toh
Fume/smoke (noun)	**Humo** Oo-moh
Intensive care	**Cuidado intensivo** Kwih-**dah**-doh een-tehn-**see**-boh

Cough

Tos

Tohs

When did the cough start?	¿Cuándo empezó la tos? **Kwahn**-doh ehm-peh-**soh** lah tohs?
It has been __ hours.	Hace __ horas. Ah-seh **oh**-rahs
__ days	__ días **dee**-ahs
__ weeks	__ semanas seh-**mah**-nahs
Does he / she have a dry cough?	¿Tiene la tos seca? **Tee-eh**-neh lah tohs seh-kah?
Does he / she have phlegm?	¿Tiene flema? **Tee-eh**-neh **fleh**-mah?
What color is it?	¿De qué color es? Deh **keh** koh-**lohr** ehs?
__ White	__ Blanca **Blahn**-kah
__ Yellow	__ Amarilla Ah-mah-**ree**-yah
__ Green	__ Verde **Behr**-deh
Have you noticed blood in the phlegm?	¿Ha notado sangre en la flema? Ah noh-**tah**-doh **sahn**-greh ehn lah **fleh**-mah?

Does the phlegm have blood streaks?

¿Tiene manchas de sangre la flema?
Tee-eh-neh **mahn**-chahs deh **sahn**-greh lah **fleh**-mah?

Does he / she have a barking cough?

¿Tiene tos perruna?
Tee-eh-neh tohs peh-**rhoo**-nah?

Does he / she have fever?

¿Tiene fiebre?
Tee-eh-neh **fee-eh**-breh?

Does he / she have difficulty breathing?

¿Tiene dificultad para respirar?
Tee-eh-neh dee-fee-kool-**tahd** pah-rah rehs-pee-**rahr?**

Does he / she have asthma?

¿Tiene asma?
Tee-eh-neh **ahs**-mah?

(If he / she has asthma refer to the chapter on asthma.)

Does he / she have allergies?

¿Tiene alergias?
Tee-eh-neh ah-**lehr-hee**-ahs?

Does he / she have a runny nose?

¿Tiene la nariz escurriendo?
Tee-eh-neh lah nah-**rees** ehs-koo-ree-**ehn**-doh?

Does he / she have a sore throat?

¿Tiene dolor de garganta?
Tee-eh-neh doh-**lohr** deh gahr-**gahn**-tah?

Is he / she taking medication for cough?

¿Está tomando medicina para la tos?
Ehs-**tah** toh-**mahn**-doh meh-dee-**see**-nah pah-rah lah tohs?

___ Cough syrup

___ Jarabe de la tos
Ha-**rah**-beh deh lah tohs

___ Antibiotics

___ Antibióticos
Ahn-tee-bee-**oh**-tee-kohs

Has he / she lost weight?

¿Ha perdido peso?
Ah pehr-**dee**-doh **peh**-soh?

Does he / she have night sweats?

¿Suda durante la noche?
Soo-dah doo-**rahn**-teh lah **noh**-cheh?

Has he / she had contact with someone with tuberculosis?

¿Ha tenido contacto con una persona con tuberculosis?
Ah teh-**nee**-doh kohn-**tahk**-toh kohn **oo**-nah pehr-**soh**-nah kohn too-**behr**-koo-**loh**-sees?

Has he / she had the skin test for tuberculosis?

¿Ha tenido el examen de la piel para la tuberculosis?
Ah teh-**nee**-doh ehl eg-**sah**-mehn deh lah pee-ehl pah-rah lah too-**behr**-koo-**loh**-sees?

When?

¿Cuándo?
Kwahn-doh?

What was the result of the test?

¿Cuál fué el resultado de la prueba?
Kwahl fweh ehl reh-sool-**tah**-doh deh lah **proo-eh**-bah?

___ Positive

___ Positivo
Poh-see-**tee**-boh

___ Negative

___ Negativo
Neh-gah-**tee**-boh

___ Does not know

___ No sabe
Noh sah-beh

Common Terms During the Exam for Cough

Breathe deeply.	Respire profundo. Rehs-**pee**-reh proh-**foon**-doh.
Cough (command).	Tosa. **Toh**-sah.
He / she needs a chest X-ray.	Él / ella necesita una radiografía del pecho. Ehl / eh-yah neh-seh-**see**-tah-ah **oo**-nah **rah**-dee-oh-grah-**fee-ah** dehl **peh**-choh.
He / she needs intravenous antibiotics.	Él / ella necesita antibióticos intravenosos. Ehl / eh-yah neh-seh-**see**-tah ahn-tee-bee-**oh**-tee-kohs een-trah-beh-**noh**-sohs.
He / she has pneumonia.	Él / ella tiene pulmonía. Ehl / eh-yah **tee-eh**-neh pool-moh-**nee-ah.**
He / she has the flu.	Él / ella tiene gripa. Ehl / eh-yah **tee-eh**-neh **gree**-pah.
He / she has asthma.	Él / ella tiene asma. Ehl / eh-yah **tee-eh**-neh **ahs**-mah.
Your child needs the tuberculosis test today.	Su niño / niña necesita la prueba de la tuberculosis hoy. Soo **nee**-nyoh / **nee**-nyah neh-seh-**see**-tah lah **proo-eh**-bah deh lah too-**behr**-koo-**loh**-sees oy.

We need to admit him / her.

Necesitamos internarlo (la).
Neh-seh-see-**tah**-mohs **een**-tehr-**nahr**-loh (lah).

Discharge Instructions for Cough

Return to the hospital if he / she has . . .

Regrese al hospital si tiene . . .
Reh-**greh**-seh ahl **ohs**-pee-tahl see **tee-eh**-neh . . .

___ shortness of breath

___ **falta de aire**
fahl-tah deh ay-reh

___ persistent fever / vomiting

___ **fiebre persistente / vómito persistente**
fee-eh-breh pehr-sees-**tehn**-teh / **boh**-mee-toh pehr-sees-**tehn**-teh

Return to the hospital or go see your doctor to read the tuberculosis skin test in two days.

Regrese al hospital o vea a su médico para revisarle el examen de la tuberculosis en dos días.
Reh-**greh**-seh ahl **ohs**-pee-tahl oh beh-ah ah soo **meh**-dee-koh pah-rah reh-bee-**sahr**-le ehl eg-**sah**-mehn deh lah too-**behr**-koo-**loh**-sees ehn dohs **dee**-ahs.

Give him / her the antibiotics every ___ hours.

Déle el antibiótico cada ___ horas.
Deh-leh ehl ahn-tee-bee-**oh**-tee-koh kah-dah ___ **oh**-rahs.

Chest Pain

Dolor de Pecho

Doh-**lohr** deh **peh**-choh

Where does he / she have the pain?

¿Dónde tiene el dolor?
Dohn-deh **tee-eh**-neh ehl doh-**lohr?**

Does he / she have pain in the left side of the chest?

¿Tiene dolor en el lado izquierdo del pecho?
Tee-eh-neh doh-**lohr** ehn ehl lah-doh ees-**kee-ehr**-doh dehl **peh**-choh?

Does he / she have pain in the right side of the chest?

¿Tiene dolor en el lado derecho del pecho?
Tee-eh-neh doh-**lohr** ehn ehl lah-doh deh-**reh**-choh?

Does he / she have pain in the middle of the chest?

¿Tiene dolor en medio del pecho?
Tee-eh-neh doh-**lohr** ehn meh-dee-oh dehl **peh**-choh?

Does he / she have pain now?

¿Tiene dolor ahora?
Tee-eh-neh doh-**lohr** ah-**oh**-rah?

How is the pain?

¿Cómo es el dolor?
Koh-moh ehs ehl do-**lohr**?

___ Sharp

___ Agudo
Ah-**goo**-doh

___ Strong

___ Fuerte
Fwehr-teh

___ Burning

___ Ardor
Ahr-**dohr**

___ Pressure-like

___ Como presión
Koh-moh preh-**see-ohn**

___ Like a knife

___ Como cuchillo
Koh-moh koo-**chee**-yoh

___ Sticking (like a needle)

___ Piquetes (como aguja)
Pee-**keh**-tehs (**koh**-moh
ah-**goo**-hah)

How long does the pain last?

¿Cuánto tiempo le dura el
dolor?
Kwahn-toh **tee-ehm**-poh leh
doo-rah ehl doh-**lohr?**

___ seconds

___ segundos
seh-**goon**-dohs

___ minutes

___ minutos
mee-**noo**-tohs

___ hours

___ horas
oh-rahs

___ constant

___ constante
kohns-**tahn**-teh

Does the pain come and go?

¿Le va y viene el dolor?
Leh bah ee bee-eh-neh ehl
doh-**lohr?**

Does the pain go to . . .

¿Le va el dolor a . . .
Leh bah ehl doh-**lohr** a . . .

___ the shoulder

___ el hombro
ehl **ohm**-broh

___ the neck

___ el cuello
ehl **kweh**-yoh

___ the back

___ la espalda
lah ehs-**pahl**-dah

___ the abdomen

___ el abdomen
ehl ab-**doh**-mehn

Does he / she have shortness of breath?

¿Tiene falta de aire?
Tee-eh-neh fahl-tah deh ay-reh?

Does it hurt more when he / she takes a deep breath?

¿Le duele más cuando respira profundo?
Leh dweh-leh mahs **kwahn**-doh rehs-**pee**-rah proh-**foon**-doh?

Does he / she have a cough?

¿Tiene tos?
Tee-eh-neh tohs?

Does it hurt more when he / she coughs?

¿Le duele más cuando tose?
Leh dweh-leh mahs **kwahn**-doh **toh**-seh?

Does he / she have fever?

¿Tiene fiebre?
Tee-eh-neh **fee-eh**-breh?

Does he / she have vomiting?

¿Tiene vómito?
Tee-eh-neh **boh**-mee-toh?

Does he / she have abdominal pain?

¿Tiene dolor abdominal?
Tee-eh-neh doh-**lohr** abh-doh-mee-**nahl?**

Did someone hit him / her in the chest?

¿Alguien le pegó en el pecho?
Ahl-gee-ehn leh peh-**goh** ehn ehl **peh**-choh?

Did he / she fall?

¿Se cayó?
Seh kah-**yoh?**

What was he / she doing when the pain started?	¿Qué estaba haciendo cuando empezó el dolor? **Keh** ehs-**tah**-bah ah-see-**ehn**-doh **kwahn**-doh ehm-peh-**soh** ehl doh-**lohr?**

___ Running	___ Corriendo Koh-rhee-**ehn**-doh
___ Talking	___ Hablando Ah-**blahn**-doh
___ Eating	___ Comiendo Koh-mee-**ehn**-doh
___ Playing	___ Jugando Hoo-**gahn**-doh
___ Nothing	___ Nada Nah-dah

Does he / she have asthma?	¿Tiene asma? **Tee-eh**-neh **ahs**-mah?
Does he / she have more pain when he / she runs or plays sports?	¿Tiene más dolor cuando corre o juega deportes? **Tee-eh**-neh mahs doh-**lohr** **kwahn**-doh koh-reh oh hoo-eh-gah deh-**pohr**-tehs?
Does it hurt more when he / she moves his / her arms?	¿Le duele más cuando mueve sus brazos? Leh dweh-leh mahs **kwahn**-doh **mweh**-beh soos **brah**-sohs?
Did you give him / her medicine for the pain?	¿Le dió medicina para el dolor? Leh dee-**oh** meh-dee-**see**-nah pah-rah ehl doh-**lohr?**

___ Tylenol

___ Tylenol
Tay-leh-nohl

___ Advil

___ Advil
Ad-beel

___ Motrin

___ Motrin
Moh-treen

Common Terms During the Exam for Chest Pain

Show me where you have the pain.

Muéstreme donde tiene el dolor.
Mwehs-treh-meh **dohn**-deh **tee-eh**-neh ehl doh-**lohr.**

Does it hurt when I press on your chest?

¿Le duele cuando le oprimo el pecho?
Leh dweh-leh **kwahn**-doh leh oh-**pree**-moh ehl **peh**-choh?

Take a deep breath.

Respire profundo.
Rehs-**pee**-reh proh-**foon**-doh.

He / she needs an electrocardiogram.

Él / ella necesita un electrocardiograma.
Ehl / eh-yah neh-seh-**see**-tah oon eh-lek-troh-kahr-deeh-oh-**grah**-mah.

He / she needs a chest X-ray.

Él / ella necesita una radiografía del pecho.
Ehl / eh-yah neh-seh-**see**-tah **oo**-nah **rah**-dee-oh-grah-**fee-ah** dehl **peh**-choh.

He / she needs an echocardiogram.

Él / ella necesita un ecocardiograma.
Ehl / eh-yah neh-seh-**see**-tah oon eh-koh-kahr-dee-oh-**grah**-mah.

He / she has pneumonia.

Él / ella tiene pulmonía.
Ehl / eh-yah **tee-eh**-neh pool-moh-**neeh-ah.**

He / she has a pneumothorax (collapsed lung).

Él / ella tiene un neumotórax (colapso del pulmón).
Ehl / eh-yah **tee-eh**-neh oon neh-oo-moh-**toh**-raks (koh-**lahp**-soh dehl pool-**mohn**).

He / she has pericarditis.

Él / ella tiene pericarditis.
Ehl / eh-yah **tee-eh**-neh peh-ree-kahr-**dee**-tees.

Pericarditis is an inflammation of the heart sac.

Pericarditis es inflamación del saco del corazón.
Peh-ree-kahr-dee-tees ehs een-flah-mah-**see-ohn**-dehl sah-koh dehl koh-rah-**sohn.**

He / she has pleurisy.

Él / ella tiene pleuresía.
Ehl / eh-yah **tee-eh**-neh pleh-oo-reh-**see-ah.**

Pleurisy is an inflammation of the lung sac.

Pleuresía es inflamación del saco del pulmón.
Pleh-oo-re-**see-ah** ehs een-flah-mah-**see-ohn** dehl sah-koh dehl pool-**mohn.**

His / her heart is fine.

Su corazón está bien.
Soo koh-rah-**sohn** ehs-**tah** bee-ehn.

He / she needs antibiotics.

Él / ella necesita antibióticos.
Ehl / eh-yah neh-seh-**see**-tah ahn-tee-bee-**oh**-tee-kohs.

He / she needs anti-inflammatory medicine.

Él / ella necesita medicina anti-inflamatoria.
Ehl / eh-yah neh-seh-**see**-tah meh-dee-**see**-nah ahn-tee-een-flah-mah-**toh**-ree-ah.

He / she has musculoskeletal pain.

Él / ella tiene dolor muscular.
Ehl / eh-yah **tee-eh**-neh doh-**lohr** moos-koo-**lahr.**

He / she has a heart mumur.

Él / ella tiene un soplo en el corazón.
Ehl / eh-yah **tee-eh**-neh oon soh-ploh ehn ehl koh-rah-**sohn.**

He / she has heart failure.

Él / ella tiene insuficiencia cardíaca.
Ehl / eh-yah **tee-eh**-neh een-soo-fee-see-**ehn**-see-ah kahr-**dee**-ah-kah.

Discharge Instructions for Chest Pain

Give him / her antibiotics every ___ hours.

Déle antibióticos cada ___ horas.
Deh-leh ahn-tee-bee-**oh**-tee-kohs kah dah ___ **oh**-rahs.

Give him / her ibuprofen every ___ hours.

Déle ibuprofen cada ___ horas.
Deh-leh ee-boo-proh-fehn kah-dah ___ **oh**-rahs.

Return to the hospital if he / she has . . .

Regrese al hospital si el / ella tiene . . .
Reh-**greh**-seh ahl **ohs**-pee-tahl see ehl / eh-yah **tee-eh**-neh . . .

___ difficulty breathing

___ **dificultad para respirar**
dee-fee-kool-**tahd** pah-rah rehs-pee-**rahr**

___ shortness of breath

___ **falta de aire**
fahl-tah deh ay-reh

___ fever

___ **fiebre**
fee-eh-breh

___ worsening chest pain

___ **peor dolor de pecho**
peh-ohr doh-**lohr** deh **peh**-choh

PART **C**

Gastrointestine

Vomiting

Vómito
Boh-mee-toh

When did he / she start vomiting?

¿Cuándo empezó a vomitar?
Kwahn-doh ehm-peh-**soh** ah boh-mee-**tahr?**

___ Today

___ Hoy
Oy

___ Yesterday

___ Ayer
Ah-**yehr**

It has been ___ days.

Hace ___ días.
Ah-seh **dee**-ahs.

What color is the emesis?

¿De qué color es el vómito?
Deh **keh** koh-**lohr** ehs ehl **boh**-mee-toh?

___ Green

___ Verde
Behr-deh

___ Yellow

___ Amarillo
Ah-mah-**ree**-yoh

___ Dark brown

___ Café obscuro
Kah-**feh** obs-**koo**-roh

___ Red

___ Rojo
Roh-ho

Have you noticed blood in the vomit?

¿Ha notado sangre en el vómito?
Ah noh-**tah**-doh **sahn**-greh ehn ehl **boh**-mee-toh?

How many times a day does he / she vomit?

¿Cuántas veces vomita al día?
Kwahn-tahs **beh**-sehs boh-**mee**-tah ahl **dee**-ah?

When was the last time he / she vomited?

¿Cuándo fué la última vez que vomitó?
Kwahn-doh **fweh** lah **ool**-tee-mah behs **keh** boh-mee-**toh?**

___ hours

hace ___ horas
ah-seh   oh-rahs

___ days

___ días
dee-ahs

Does he / she have diarrhea?

¿Tiene diarrea?
Tee-eh-neh dee-ah-**rhe-ah?**

How many times a day does he / she have diarrhea?

¿Cuántas veces al día tiene diarrea?
Kwahn-tahs **beh**-sehs ahl **dee**-ah **tee-eh**-neh dee-ah-**rhe-ah?**

Have you noticed blood in the diarrhea?

¿Ha notado sangre en la diarrea?
Ah noh-**tah**-doh **sahn**-greh ehn lah dee-ah-**rhe-ah?**

Has he / she traveled outside the country recently?

¿Ha viajado fuera del país recientemente?
Ah bee-ah-**hah**-doh **fweh**-rah dehl pah-**ees** reh-see-ehn-teh-**mehn**-teh?

Where?

¿A dónde?
Ah **dohn**-deh?

Has he / she lost weight?

¿Ha perdido peso?
Ah pehr-**dee**-doh **peh**-soh?

How many pounds has he / she lost?	¿Cuántas libras ha perdido? **Kwahn**-tahs lee-brahs ah pehr-**dee**-doh?
Does he / she vomit only when you give him milk?	¿Vomita solamente cuando le da leche? Boh-**mee**-tah soh-lah-**mehn**-teh **kwahn**-doh leh dah leh-cheh?
Have you changed the formula?	¿Le ha cambiado la fórmula? Leh ah kahm-bee-**ah**-doh lah **fohr**-moo-lah?
What kind of formula does he / she take?	¿Qué clase de fórmula toma? **Keh** klah-seh deh **fohr**-moo-lah **toh**-mah?
Do you give him / her cow's milk?	¿Le da leche de vaca? Leh dah leh-cheh deh bah-kah?
Do you breastfeed?	¿Le da pecho? Leh dah **peh**-choh?
Is there another person in the house with the same symptoms?	¿Hay otra persona en casa con los mismos síntomas? Ay oh-trah pehr-**soh**-nah ehn **kah**-sah kohn lohs mees-mohs **seen**-toh-mahs?
Does he / she make tears when crying?	¿Le salen lágrimas cuando llora? Leh sah-lehn **lah**-gree-mahs **kwahn**-doh **yoh**-rah?
When was the last time he / she urinated?	¿Cuándo fué la última vez que orinó? **Kwahn**-doh **fweh** lah **ool**-tee-mah behs **keh** oh-**ree-noh?**

How many diapers did you change today?	¿Cuántos pañales le cambió hoy? **Kwahn**-tohs pah-**nyah**-lehs leh kahm-bee-**oh** oy?
How many diapers do you normally change a day?	¿Cuántos pañales le cambia normalmente al día? **Kwahn**-tohs pah-**nyah**-lehs leh kahm-bee-ah nohr-mahl-**mehn**-teh ahl **dee**-ah?
When was the last time you changed his / her diaper?	¿Cuándo fué la última vez que le cambió el pañal? **Kwahn**-doh **fweh** lah **ool**-tee-mah vehs keh leh kahm-bee-**oh** ehl pah-**nyahl?**
Is he / she active as usual?	¿Está activo (a) como usual? Ehs-**tah** ahk-**tee**-boh (bah) **koh**-moh oo-soo-ahl?
Does he / she want to play?	¿Él / ella quiere jugar? Ehl / eh-yah kee-**eh**-reh hoo-**gahr?**
Does he / she have a fever?	¿Él / ella tiene fiebre? Ehl / eh-yah **tee-eh**-neh **fee-eh**-breh?

Common Terms During the Exam for Vomiting

We need to do blood and urine tests.	Necesitamos hacerle análisis de sangre y orina. Neh-seh-see-**tah**-mos ah-**sehr**-leh ah-**nah**-lee-seehs deh **sahn**-greh ee oh-**ree**-nah.

He / she needs intravenous fluid.

Él / ella necesita suero intravenoso.
Ehl / eh-yah neh-seh-**see**-tah soo-eh-roh een-trah-beh-**noh**-soh.

We are going to admit him / her.

Vamos a internarlo (la).
Bah-mohs ah **een**-tehr-**nahr**-loh (lah).

Your child is dehydrated.

Su niño (a) está deshidratado (a).
Soo **nee**-nyoh (ah) ehs-**tah** dehs-ee-drah-**tah**-doh (ah).

He / she has a viral infection.

Él / ella tiene una infección viral.
Ehl / eh-yah **tee-eh**-neh oo-nah een-feg-**see-ohn** bee-**rahl.**

He / she does not need antibiotics.

Él / ella no necesita antibióticos.
Ehl / eh-yah noh neh-seh-**see**-tah ahn-tee-bee-**oh**-tee-kohs.

Discharge Instructions for Vomiting

Return to the hospital if . . .

Regrese al hospital si . . .
Reh-**greh**-seh ahl **ohs**-pee tahl see . . .

—— he / she continues vomiting

—— sigue vomitando
see-geh boh-mee-**tahn**-doh

—— he / she has a fever

—— él / ella tiene fiebre
ehl / eh-yah **tee-eh**-neh **fee-eh**-breh

—— he / she stops making tears or urine

—— él / ella deja de hacer lágrimas u orina
ehl / eh-yah deh-hah deh ah-sehr **lah**-gree-mahs oo oh-**ree**-nah

Don't give him / her milk for a day.

No le **dé** leche por un **día.**
Noh leh deh leh-cheh pohr oon **dee**-ah.

Give him / her Pedialyte for a day.

Déle Pedialyte por un **día.**
Deh-leh pee-dee-ah-layt pohr oon **dee**-ah.

Suspected Pyloric Stenosis

Sospecha de Estenosis Pilórica

Sohs-**peh**-chah deh ehs-teh-**noh**-sees pee-**loh**-ree-kah

When did he / she start vomiting?

¿Cuándo empezó a vomitar?
Kwahn-doh ehm-peh-**soh** ah boh-mee-**tahr?**

___ Today

___ Hoy
Oy

___ Yesterday

___ Ayer
Ah-**yehr**

It's been ___ days.

Hace ___ días.
Ah-seh **dee**-ahs.

How many times did he / she vomit today?

¿Cuántas veces vomitó hoy?
Kwahn-tahs beh-sehs boh-mee-**toh** oy?

When was the last time he / she vomited?

¿Cuándo fué la última vez que vomitó?
Kwahn-doh **fweh** lah **ool**-tee-mah behs **keh** boh-mee-**toh?**

It's been __ hours.

Hace __ horas.
Ah-seh **oh**-rahs.

__ days

__ días
dee-ahs

Does he / she vomit every time you give milk?

¿Vomita cada vez que le da leche?
Boh-**mee**-tah kah-dah behs **keh** leh dah leh-cheh?

Does he / she vomit immediately after feeding?

¿Vomita inmediatamente después de comer?
Boh-**mee**-tah een-meh-dee-ah-tah-**mehn**-teh dehs-**pwehs** deh koh-**mehr?**

Does his / her vomit shoot out in projectile form?

¿Le sale el vómito disparado en forma proyectil?
Leh sah-leh ehl **boh**-mee-toh dees-pah-**rah**-doh ehn fohr-**mah** proh-jek-**teel?**

Does it seem to you that he / she is hungry?

¿Le parece que él / ella tiene hambre?
Leh pah-**reh**-seh **keh** ehl / eh-yah **tee-eh**-neh ahm-breh?

Does he / she want to eat?

¿Quiere comer?
Kee-**eh**-reh koh-**mehr?**

Has he / she lost weight?

¿Ha perdido peso?
Ah pehr-**dee**-doh **peh**-soh?

How many pounds has he / she lost?

¿Cuántas libras ha perdido?
Kwhan-tahs lee-brahs ah pehr-**dee**-doh?

How much did he / she weigh at birth?

¿Cuánto pesó al nacer?
Kwahn-toh peh-**soh** ahl nah-sehr?

How much does he / she weigh now?

¿Cuánto pesa ahora?
Kwhan-toh **peh**-sah ah-**oh**-rah?

Does he have tears when crying?

¿Tiene lágrimas cuando llora?
Tee-eh-neh **lah**-gree-mahs **kwahn**-doh **yoh**-rah?

Did you notice blood in the vomit?

¿Notó sangre en el vómito?
Noh-**toh sahn**-greh ehn ehl **boh**-mee-toh?

What kind of formula does he / she drink?

¿Qué clase de fórmula toma?
Keh klah-seh deh **fohr**-moo-lah **toh**-mah?

Has he / she always taken that formula?

¿Ha tomado esa fórmula siempre?
Ah toh-**mah**-doh eh-sah **fohr**-moo-lah see-**ehm**-preh?

Have you changed his / her formula?

¿Le ha cambiado la fórmula?
Leh ah kahm-bee-**ah**-doh lah **fohr**-moo-lah?

Do you breastfeed him / her?

¿Le da pecho?
Leh dah **peh**-choh?

Is he / she the first born?

¿Es él / ella el primer nacido?
Ehs ehl / eh-yah ehl pree-**mehr** nah-**see**-doh?

Does he / she have another brother (sister) who had the same problem?

¿Tiene otro hermano (a) que tuvo el mismo problema?
Tee-eh-neh oh-troh ehr-**mah**-noh (nah) **keh too**-boh ehl mees-moh proh-**bleh**-mah?

Did they operate on him / her?

¿Lo operaron?
Loh oh-peh-**rah**-rohn?

Common Terms for Pyloric Stenosis

He / she needs an X-ray.

Él / ella necesita rayos equis.
Ehl / eh-yah neh-seh-**see**-tah
rha-yohs **eh**-keys.

He / she needs surgery / an
operation.

Él /ella necesita cirugía / una
operación.
Ehl / eh-yah neh-seh-**see**-tah
see-roo-**hee**-ah / **oo**-nah oh-
peh-rah-**see-ohn.**

He / she has pyloric stenosis.

Él / ella tiene estenosis
pilórica.
Ehl / eh-yah **tee-eh**-neh ehs-
teh-**noh**-sees pee-**loh**-ree-kah.

He / she needs an ultrasound.

Él / ella necesita un
ultrasonido.
Ehl / eh-yah neh-seh-**see**-tah
oon **ool**-trah-soh-**nee**-doh.

He / she needs blood tests.

Él / ella necesita pruebas de
sangre.
Ehl / eh-yah neh-seh-**see**-tah
proo-eh-bahs deh **sahn**-greh.

He / she needs intravenous
fluid.

Él / ella necesita suero
intravenoso.
Ehl / eh-yah neh-seh-**see**-tah
soo-eh-roh een-trah-beh-**noh**-
soh.

He / she needs to be
admitted.

Él / ella necesita ser internado
(a).
Ehl / eh-yah neh-seh-**see**-tah
sehr een-tehr-**nah**-doh (dah).

Diarrhea

Diarrea

Dee-ah-**rhe-ah**

For how many days does he / she have diarrhea?

¿Por cuántos días ha tenido diarrea?
Pohr **kwahn**-tohs **dee**-ahs ah teh-**nee**-doh dee-ah-**rhe-ah?**

How many times did he / she have diarrhea today?

¿Cuántas veces ha tenido diarrea hoy?
Kwahn-tahs **beh**-sehs ah teh-**nee**-doh dee-ah-**rhe-ah** oy?

What color is the diarrhea?

¿De qué color es la diarrea?
Deh **keh** koh-**lohr** ehs lah dee-ah-**rhe-ah?**

___ Yellow

___ Amarilla
Ah-mah-**ree**-yah

___ Green

___ Verde
Behr-deh

___ Black

___ Negro
Neh-groh

___ Red

___ Roja
Roh-hah

Does he / she have abdominal pain?

¿Tiene dolor abdominal?
Tee-eh-neh doh-**lohr** ab-doh-mee-**nahl?**

Have you noticed blood in the diarrhea?

¿Ha notado sangre en la diarrea?
Ah noh-**tah**-doh **sahn**-greh ehn lah dee-ah-**rhe-ah?**

Does the pain go away after he / she has diarrhea?

¿Se le quita el dolor después de tener diarrea?
Seh leh kee-tah ehl doh-**lohr** dehs-**pwehs** deh teh-**nehr** dee-ah-**rhe-ah?**

Does he / she have a fever?

¿Tiene fiebre?
Tee-eh-neh **fee-eh**-breh?

Does he / she have vomiting?

¿Tiene vómito?
Tee-eh-neh **boh**-mee-toh?

Recently, has he / she traveled outside the country or state?

¿Recientemente, ha viajado afuera del país o del estado?
Reh-see-ehn-teh-**mehn**-teh, ah bee-ah-**ha**-doh ah-**fweh**-rah dehl pah-**ees** oh dehl ehs-**tah**-doh?

Recently, has he / she eaten in fast food restaurants?

¿Recientemente, ha comido en restaurantes de comida rápida?
Reh-see-ehn-teh-**mehn**-teh, ah koh-**mee**-doh ehn rehs-tah-oo-**rahn**-tehs deh koh-**mee**-dah **rah**-pee-dah?

Is there someone living with you who has the same symptoms?

¿Hay alguien que vive con usted que tiene los mismos síntomas?
Ah-ee ahl-gee-ehn **keh** bee-beh kohn oos-**tehd keh tee-eh**-neh lohs mees-mohs **seen**-toh-mahs?

Normally, how many bowel movements does he / she have a day?

¿Normalmente, cuantas veces va al baño (obra) al día?
Nohr-mahl-**mehn**-teh, **kwahn**-tahs **beh**-sehs bah ahl **bah**-nyoh (oh-brah) ahl **dee**-ah?

When was the last time that you changed his / her diaper?

¿Cúando fué la última vez que le cambió el pañal?
Kwahn-doh **fweh** lah **ool**-tee-mah behs **keh** leh kahm-bee-**oh** ehl pah-**nyahl?**

Does he / she have tears when crying?	¿Tiene lágrimas cuando llora? **Tee-eh**-neh **lah**-gree-mahs **kwahn**-doh **yoh**-rah?

Common Terms for Diarrhea

I need to do a rectal exam.	Necesito hacerle un examen del recto. Neh-seh-**see**-toh ah-**sehr**-leh oon eg-**sah**-mehn dehl **reg**-toh.
Can you give us a stool sample?	¿Puede darnos una muestra de excremento? Pweh-deh dahr-nohs **oo**-nah **mwehs**-trah deh egs-kreh-**mehn**-toh?
He / she needs an antibiotic.	Él / ella necesita un antibiótico. Ehl / eh-yah neh-seh-**see**-tah oon ahn-tee-bee-**oh**-tee-koh.
Your child has a viral infection and doesn't need an antibiotic.	Su niño (a) tiene una infección viral y no necesita un antibiótico. Soo **nee**-nyoh (ah) **tee-eh**-neh oo-nah een-feg-**see-ohn** bee-**rahl** ee noh neh-seh-**see**-tah oon ahn-tee-bee-**oh**-tee-koh.

Discharge Instructions for Diarrhea

Return to the hospital if he / she has . . .	Regrese al hospital si él / ella tiene . . . Reh-**greh**-seh ahl **ohs**-pee-tahl see ehl / eh-yah **tee-eh**-neh . . .

___ fever

___ vomiting

___ worsening abdominal
pain

___ blood in the stools

Give him / her plenty of
fluids.

Avoid fruits and milk
products.

___ fiebre
fee-eh-breh

___ vómito
boh-mee-toh

___ peor dolor abdominal
peh-ohr doh-**lohr** ab-
doh-mee-**nahl**

___ sangre en sus heces o
excremento
sahn-greh ehn soos **eh**-
sehs oh egs-kreh-**mehn**-
toh

Déle muchos líquidos.
Deh-leh **moo**-chohs **lee**-kee-
dohs.

Evite las frutas y los productos
de leche.
Eh-**bee**-teh lahs **froo**-tahs ee
lohs proh-**dook**-tohs deh leh-
cheh.

Constipation

Estreñimiento
Ehs-treh-nyee-mee-**ehn**-toh

When was the last time he /
she had a bowel movement?

¿Cuándo fué la última vez que
obró (usó el baño)?
Kwahn-doh **fweh** lah **ool**-tee
mah behs **keh** oh-**broh** (oo-
soh ehl **bah**-nyoh)?

Normally does he / she have a bowel movement every day?

¿**Normalmente obra** todos los **días?**
Nohr-mahl-**mehn**-teh oh-brah toh-dohs lohs **dee**-ahs?

Every how many days does he / she have a bowel movement?

¿**Cada cuántos días obra?**
Kah-dah **kwahn**-tohs **dee**-ahs oh-brah?

Have you noticed if his / her stools are hard?

¿**Ha notado que sus heces son duras?**
Ah noh-**tah**-doh **keh** soos **eh**-sehs sohn **doo**-rahs?

Have you noticed blood mixed with the stools?

¿**Ha notado sangre mezclada con sus heces?**
Ah noh-**tah**-doh **sahn**-greh mehs-**klah**-dah kohn soos **eh**-sehs?

Have you noticed blood when you wipe him / her?

¿**Ha notado sangre cuando lo / la limpia?**
Ah noh-**tah**-doh **sahn**-greh **kwahn**-doh loh / lah **leem**-pee-ah?

What color are his stools?

¿**De qué color son sus heces?**
Deh **keh** koh-**lohr** sohn soos **eh**-sehs?

___ Yellow

___ **Amarillas**
Ah-mah-**ree**-yahs

___ Brown

___ **Cafés**
Kah-**fehs**

___ Green

___ **Verdes**
Behr-dehs

___ Black

___ **Negros**
Neh-grohs

Do you give him / her laxatives?

¿Le da laxantes?
Leh dah lag-**sahn**-tehs?

Does he / she complain of abdominal pain?

¿Se queja de dolor en el abdomen?
Seh **keh**-ha deh doh-**lohr** ehn ehl ab-**doh**-mehn?

Does he / she have vomiting?

¿Tiene vómito?
Tee-eh-neh **boh**-mee-toh?

Does he / she have a fever?

¿Tiene fiebre?
Tee-eh-neh **fee-eh**-breh?

Did you change his / her formula?

¿Le cambió la formula?
Leh kahm-bee-**oh** lah **fohr**-moo-lah?

Does he / she eat fresh fruits?

¿Come frutas frescas?
Koh-meh **froo**-tahs **frehs**-kahs?

Does he / she eat fresh vegetables?

¿Come vegetales frescos?
Koh-meh beh-heh-**tah**-lehs **frehs**-kohs?

Do you give him / her water between feedings?

¿Le da agua entre comidas?
Leh dah **ah**-gwah ehn-treh koh-**mee**-dahs?

Common Terms for Constipation

I need to do a rectal exam.

¿Necesito hacerle un examen del recto.
Neh-seh-**see**-toh ah-**sehr**-leh oon eg-**sah**-mehn dehl **reg**-toh.

He / she has a fecal impaction.

Él / ella está tapado / a con heces.
Ehl / eh-yah ehs-**tah** tah-pah-doh / dah kohn **eh**-sehs.

We need to give him / her an enema.	Necesitamos darle un enema. Neh-seh-see-**tah**-mohs dahr-leh oon eh-neh-mah.

Discharge Instructions for Constipation

Return to the hospital if he / she has . . .	Regrese al hospital si él / ella tiene . . . Reh-**greh**-seh ahl **ohs**-pee-tahl see ehl / eh-yah **tee-eh**-neh . . .
___ fever	___ fiebre **fee-eh**-breh
___ vomiting	___ vómito **boh**-mee-toh
___ worsening abdominal pain	___ peor dolor abdominal peh-ohr doh-**lohr** ab-doh-mee-**nahl**
___ blood in the stools	___ sangre en sus heces (excremento) **sahn**-greh ehn soos **eh**-sehs (egs-kreh-**mehn**-toh)
Do not use laxatives.	No use laxantes. Noh oo-seh lag-**sahn**-tehs.
Give him / her more fruits and vegetables.	Déle más frutas y vegetales. **Deh**-leh mahs **froo**-tahs ee beh-heh-**tah**-lehs.

Rectal Bleeding

Sangrado Rectal

When did **you notice the** blood?

¿**Cuándo** notó la sangre?
Kwahn-doh noh-**toh** lah **sahn**-greh?

___ Today

___ **Hoy**
Oy

___ Days ago

Hace ___ **días**
Ah-seh **dee**-ahs

Is the blood mixed with stools?

¿**Está mezclada la sangre con el excremento?**
Ehs-**tah** mehs-**klah**-dah lah **sahn**-greh kohn ehl egs-kreh-**mehn**-toh?

Are the stools streaked with blood?

¿**Está manchado con sangre el** excremento?
Ehs-**tah** mahn-**chah**-doh kohn **sahn**-greh ehl egs-kreh-**mehn**-toh?

Do you notice blood when you wipe him / her?

¿Usted nota sangre **cuando** lo / la limpia?
Oos-**tehd** noh-tah **sahn**-greh **kwahn**-doh loh / lah **leem**-pee-ah?

Is there bleeding each time he / she defecates?

¿Hay sangrado cada vez que obra / defeca?
Ay sahn-grah-doh kah-dah behs **keh** oh-brah / deh-**feh**-kah?

What color is the blood?

¿De qué color es la sangre?
Deh **keh** koh-**lohr** ehs lah
sahn-greh?

___ Red

___ Roja
Roh-hah

___ Brown

___ Café
Kah-**feh**

___ Maroon

___ Marrón
Mah-**rhon**

Is he / she constipated?

¿Está estreñido (a)?
Ehs-**tah** ehs-treh-**nyeh**-doh
(ah)?

When was the last time that
he / she defecated?

¿Cuándo fué la última vez que
obró / defecó?
Kwahn-doh **fweh** lah **ool**-tee-
mah behs **keh** oh-**broh** / deh-
feh-**koh?**

___ Today

___ Hoy
Oy

___ Days ago

Hace ___ días
Ah-seh   **dee**-ahs

Were his / her stools hard?

¿Eran duras sus heces?
Eh-rahn **doo**-rahs soos **eh**-
sehs?

Were his / her stools of
normal consistency?

¿Eran de consistencia normal
sus heces?
Eh-rahn deh kohn-sees-**tehn**-
see-ah nohr-**mahl** soos **eh**-
sehs?

Does he / she defecate every
day?

¿Obra / defeca todos los días?
Oh-brah / deh-**feh**-kah toh-
dohs lohs **dee**-ahs?

Common Terms for Rectal Bleeding

I need to do a rectal exam.	Necesito hacerle un examen del recto. Neh-seh-**see**-toh ah-**sehr**-leh oon eg-**sah**-mehn dehl **reg**-toh.
He / she is constipated.	Está estreñido (a). Ehs-**tah** ehs-treh-**nyeh**-doh (ah).
He / she has an anal fissure.	Él / ella tiene una fisura anal. Ehl / eh-yah **tee-eh**-neh oo-nah fee-**soo**-rah ah-**nahl.**

Discharge Instructions for Rectal Bleeding

Return to the hospital if he / she has . . .	Regrese al hospital si tiene . . . Reh-**greh**-seh ahl **ohs**-pee-tahl see **tee-eh**-neh . . .
___ more bleeding	___ más sangrado mahs sahn-**grah**-doh
___ fever	___ fiebre **fee-eh**-breh
___ abdominal pain	___ dolor abdominal doh-**lohr** ab-doh-mee-**nahl**
___ vomiting	___ vómito **boh**-mee-toh
Give him / her water between feedings.	Déle agua entre las comidas. **Deh**-leh **ah**-gwah ehn-treh lahs koh-**mee**-dahs.

Do not give him / her laxatives.

No le dé laxantes.
Noh leh deh lag-**sahn**-tehs.

Abdominal Pain

Dolor Abdominal

Doh-**lohr** ab-doh-mee-**nahl**

Show me where the pain started.

Enséñeme dónde empezó el dolor.
Ehn-**seh**-nyeh-meh **dohn**-deh ehm-peh-**soh** ehl doh-**lohr.**

Show me with one finger where he / she has the pain.

Enséñeme con un solo dedo dónde tiene el dolor.
Ehn-**seh**-nyeh-meh kohn oon soh-loh **deh**-doh **dohn**-deh **tee-eh**-neh ehl doh-**lohr.**

For how many days or hours has he / she had pain?

¿Por cuántos días u horas ha tenido dolor?
Pohr **kwahn**-tohs **dee**-ahs oo **oh**-rahs ah teh-**nee**-doh ehl doh-**lohr?**

Is the pain constant?

¿Es el dolor constante?
Ehs ehl doh-**lohr** kohns-**tahn**-teh?

Does the pain come and go?

¿Le va y viene el dolor?
Leh bah ee bee-eh-neh ehl doh-**lohr?**

Does the pain go to the back?

¿Le va el dolor a la espalda?
Leh bah ehl doh-**lohr** ah lah ehs-**pahl**-dah?

Does the pain go to the testicles?

¿Le va el dolor a los testículos?
Leh bah ehl doh-**lohr** ah lohs tehs-**tee-koo**-lohs?

Does the pain go to the groin?	¿Le va el dolor a la ingle? Leh bah ehl doh-**lohr** ah lah **een**-gleh?
Does the pain go to the bladder?	¿Le va el dolor a la vejiga? Leh bah ehl doh-**lohr** ah lah beh-**hee**-gah?
Does he / she have vomiting?	¿Tiene vómito? **Tee-eh**-neh **boh**-mee-toh?
Did the vomiting start first?	¿Empezó primero el vómito? Ehm-peh-**soh** pree-**meh**-roh ehl **boh**-mee-toh?
Did the pain start first?	¿Empezó primero el dolor? Ehm-peh-**soh** pree-**meh**-roh ehl doh-**lohr?**
How many times has he / she vomited today?	¿Cuántas veces ha vomitado hoy? **Kwahn**-tahs **beh**-sehs ah boh-mee-**tah**-doh oy?
Does he / she have diarrhea?	¿Tiene diarrea? **Tee-eh**-neh dee-ah-**rhe-ah?**
How many times did he / she have diarrhea today?	¿Cuántas veces ha tenido diarrea hoy? **Kwahn**-tahs **beh**-sehs ah teh-**nee**-doh dee-ah-**rhe-ah** oy?
What color is the diarrhea?	¿De qué color es la diarrea? Deh **keh** koh-**lohr** ehs lah dee-ah-**rhe-ah?**
___ Red	___ Roja **Roh**-ha
___ Yellow	___ Amarilla Ah-mah-**ree**-yah

___ Green

___ Black

When was the last time he / she went to the bathroom?

Does he / she have a fever?

For how many days has he / she had fever?

Does it burn when he / she urinates?

Does it hurt when he / she urinates?

Is he / she urinating more than usual?

Does he / she have blood in the urine?

When was the last time he / she ate?

___ Verde
Behr-deh

___ Negro
Neh-groh

¿Cuándo fué la última vez que fué al baño?
Kwahn-doh **fweh** lah **ool**-tee-mah behs **keh fweh** ahl **bah**-nyoh?

¿Tiene fiebre?
Tee-eh-neh **fee-eh**-breh?

¿Por cuántos días ha tenido fiebre?
Pohr **kwahn**-tohs **dee**-ahs ah teh-**nee**-doh **fee-eh**-breh?

¿Le arde cuándo orina?
Leh ahr-deh **kwahn**-doh oh-**ree**-nah?

¿Le duele cuándo orina?
Leh dweh-leh **kwahn**-doh oh-**ree**-nah?

¿Esta orinando más de lo normal?
Ehs-**tah** oh-ree-**nahn**-doh mahs deh loh nohr-**mahl?**

¿Tiene sangre en la orina?
Tee-eh-neh **sahn**-greh ehn lah oh-**ree**-nah?

¿Cuándo fué la última vez que comió?
Kwahn-doh **fweh** lah **ool**-tee-mah behs **keh** koh-mee-**oh?**

Is he / she hungry?

¿Tiene hambre?
Tee-eh-neh ahm-breh?

Common Terms During the Exam for Abdominal Pain

I am going to examine his / her abdomen.

Voy a examinar su abdomen.
Boy ah eg-sah-mee-**nahr** soo ab-**doh**-mehn.

Bend your knees.

Doble las rodillas.
Doh-bleh lahs roh-**dee**-yhahs.

Do you have pain here?

¿Tiene dolor aquí?
Tee-eh-neh doh-**lohr** ah-**kee?**

We need to do blood and urine tests.

Necesitamos hacerle pruebas de sangre y orina.
Neh-seh-see-**tah**-mohs ah-**sehr**-leh **proo-eh**-bahs deh **sahn**-greh ee oh-**ree**-nah.

I need to do a rectal exam.

Necesito hacerle un examen del recto.
Neh-seh-**see**-toh ah-**sehr**-leh oon eg-**sah**-mehn dehl **reg**-toh.

I need to do a genital exam.

Necesito hacerle un examen genital.
Neh-seh-**see**-toh ah-**sehr**-leh oon eg-**sah**-mehn he-nee-**tahl.**

I need to do a pelvic exam.

Necesito hacerle un examen pélvico.
Neh-seh-**see**-toh ah-**sehr**-leh oon eg-**sah**-mehn **pehl**-bee-koh.

We are going to get radiographs.	Vamos a sacarle radiografías. Bah-mohs ah sah-**kahr**-leh **rah**-dee-oh-grah-**fee-ahs.**
He / she needs an ultrasound.	Él / ella necesita un ultrasonido. Ehl / eh-yah neh-seh-**see**-tah oon **ool**-trah-soh-**nee**-doh.
He / she needs an operation.	Él / ella necesita una operación. Ehl / eh-yah neh-seh-**see**-tah **oo**-nah oh-peh-rah-**see-ohn.**
He / she has appendicitis.	Él / ella tiene apendicitis. Ehl / eh-yah **tee-eh**-neh ah-pehn-dee-**see**-tees.
He / she has a viral infection.	Él / ella tiene una infección viral. Ehl / eh-yah **tee-eh**-neh oo-nah een-feg-**see-ohn** bee-**rahl.**

Discharge Instructions for Abdominal Pain

Return to the hospital if . . .	Regrese al hospital si . . . Reh-**greh**-seh ahl **ohs**-pee-tahl see . . .
___ he / she has a fever.	___ él / ella tiene fiebre. ehl/eh-yah **tee-eh**-neh **fee-eh**-breh.
___ the pain is worse or the pain increases.	___ el dolor se pone peor o aumenta. ehl doh-**lohr** seh poh-neh peh-**ohr** oh ah-oo-**mehn**-tah.

___ he / she has vomiting.

___ él /ella tiene vómito.
Ehl / eh-yah **tee-eh**-neh
boh-mee-toh.

Crying / Colic

Llorando / Cólico

Yoh-rahn-doh / **Koh**-lee-koh

When did the baby start crying?

¿Cuándo empezó a llorar el bebé?
Kwahn-doh ehm-peh-**soh** ah
yoh-rahr ehl beh-**beh?**

___ It has been ___ hours

Hace ___ horas
Ah-seh **oh**-rahs

___ days.

___ días.
dee-ahs.

Does he / she bend his knees when he cries?

¿Dobla sus rodillas cuando llora?
Doh-blah soos roh-**dee**-yhahs
kwahn-doh **yoh**-rah?

Are there periods when the baby stops crying?

¿Hay periodos cuando el bebé deja de llorar?
Ah-ee peh-ree-oh-dohs
kwahn-doh ehl beh-**beh** deh-
hah deh yoh-**rahr?**

Does he / she cry constantly?

¿Llora constantemente?
Yoh-rah kohns-tahn-teh-**mehn**-
teh?

Does he / she cry more at night?

¿Llora más en la noche?
Yoh-rah mahs ehn lah **noh**-
cheh?

Does he / she cry when he / she . . .	¿Llora cuando va a . . . **Yoh**-rah **kwahn**-doh bah ah . . .
___ urinates	___ orinar oh-ree-nahr
___ defecates	___ obrar oh-brahr

Does he / she stop crying after defecating?

¿Deja de llorar despues de obrar?
Deh-ha deh yoh-**rahr** dehs-**pwehs** deh oh-**brahr?**

Does he / she stop crying after passing gas?

¿Deja de llorar después de pasar gas?
Deh-ha deh yoh-**rahr** dehs-**pwehs** deh pah-**sahr** gahs?

Does he / she stop crying after you feed him / her?

¿Deja de llorar después de darle de comer?
Deh-ha deh yoh-**rahr** dehs-**pwehs** deh dahr-leh deh koh-**mehr?**

Is he / she constipated?

¿Está estreñido (a)?
Ehs-**tah** ehs-treh-**nyeh**-doh (dah)?

Have you noticed blood in his / her stools?

¿Ha notado sangre en sus heces?
Ah noh-**tah**-doh **sahn**-greh ehn soos **eh**-sehs?

Does he / she have diarrhea?

¿Tiene diarrea?
Tee-eh-neh dee-ah-**rhe-ah?**

Does he / she have vomiting?

¿Tiene vómito?
Tee-eh-neh **boh**-mee-toh?

Does he / she have fever?	¿Tiene fiebre? **Tee-eh**-neh **fee-eh**-breh?
Is he / she pulling his / her ears?	¿Se está tirando / jalando las orejas? Seh ehs-**tah** tee-**rahn**-doh / ha-**lahn**-doh lahs oh-**reh**-has?
Can you console him / her?	¿Puede consolarlo (la)? Pweh-deh kohn-soh-**lahr**-loh (lah)?
Is he / she taking the bottle?	¿Está tomando la botella? Ehs-**tah** toh-**mahn**-doh lah boh-**teh**-yhah?
Have you changed his / her formula?	¿Ha cambiado su fórmula? Ah kahm-bee-**ah**-doh soo **fohr**-moo-lah?
Is he / she teething?	¿Le están saliendo los dientes? Leh ehs-**tahn** sah-lee-**ehn**-doh lohs dee-**ehn**-tehs?

Common Terms for Crying / Colic

Your baby has an ear infection.	Su bebé tiene una infección en los oídos. Soo beh-**beh tee-eh**-neh oo-nah een-feg-**see-ohn** ehn lohs oh-**ee**-dohs.
Your baby has colic.	Su bebé tiene cólico. Soo beh-**beh tee-eh**-neh **koh**-lee-koh.
Your baby has an infection of the urine.	Su bebé tiene una infección de la orina. Soo beh-**beh tee-eh**-neh oo-nah een-feg-**see-ohn** deh lah oh-**ree**-nah.

Your baby is constipated.	Su bebé está estreñido (a).
	Soo beh-**beh** ehs-**tah** ehs-treh-**nyeh**-doh (dah).

Discharge Instructions for Crying / Colic

Return to the hospital if . . .
Regrese al hospital si . . .
Reh-**greh**-seh ahl **ohs**-pee-tahl see . . .

__ the baby has a fever

__ el bebé tiene fiebre
ehl beh-**beh tee-eh**-neh **fee-eh**-breh

__ the baby has vomiting

__ el bebé tiene vómito
ehl beh-**beh tee-eh**-neh **boh**-mee-toh

__ there is blood in the baby's stool

__ hay sangre en las heces del bebé
ah-ee **sahn**-greh ehn lahs **eh**-sehs dehl beh-**beh**

Jaundice

Ictericia

Eek-teh-ree-see-ah

How long has his / her skin been yellow?

¿Por cuánto tiempo tiene la piel amarilla?
Pohr **kwahn**-toh **tee-ehm**-poh **tee-eh**-neh lah pee-ehl ah-mah-**ree**-yah?

Does he / she have abdominal pain?

¿Tiene dolor abdominal?
Tee-eh-neh doh-**lohr** ab-doh-mee-**nahl?**

Does he / she have vomiting?	¿Tiene vómito? **Tee-eh**-neh **boh**-mee-toh?
Does he / she have fever?	¿Tiene fiebre? **Tee-eh**-neh **fee-eh**-breh?
What color is his / her urine?	¿De qué color es su orina? Deh **keh** koh-**lohr** ehs soo oh-**ree**-nah?
___ Clear yellow	___ Amarilla clara Ah-mah-**ree**-yah **klah**-rah
___ Dark yellow	___ Amarilla obscura Ah-mah-**ree**-yah ohbs-**koo**-rah
___ Coca-cola color	___ Color de coca-cola Koh-**lohr** deh koh-kah koh-lah
What color are his / her stools?	¿De qué color son sus excrementos? Deh **keh** koh-**lohr** sohn soos egs-kreh-**mehn**-tohs?
___ Clear	___ Claros **Klah**-rohs
___ Black	___ Negros **Neh**-grohs
___ Brown	___ Cafés Kah-**fehs**
Is he / she bleeding from anywhere?	¿Tiene sangrado de algún lugar? **Tee-eh**-neh sahn-**grah**-doh deh ahl-**goon** loo-**gahr?**

Has he / she traveled outside the country recently?	¿Ha viajado afuera del país recientemente? Ah bee-ah-**hah**-doh ah-**fweh**-rah dehl pah-**ees** reh-see-ehn-teh-**mehn**-teh?
Where did he / she go?	¿A dónde fué? Ah **dohn**-deh **fweh?**
Has he / she received a blood transfusion recently?	¿Ha recibido una transfusión de sangre recientemente? Ah reh-see-**bee**-doh oo-nah trahns-foo-**see-ohn** deh **sahn**-greh reh-see-ehn-teh-**mehn**-teh?
Has he / she received the hepatitis vaccine?	¿Ha recibido la vacuna de la hepatitis? Ah reh-see-**bee**-doh lah bah-**koo**-nah deh lah eh-pah-**tee**-tees?
Has he / she had contact with a person with hepatitis?	¿Ha tenido contacto con una persona con hepatitis? Ah teh-**nee**-doh kohn-**tahk**-toh kohn **oo**-nah pehr-**soh**-nah kohn eh-pah-**tee**-tees?
Does he / she eat in fast food restaurants?	¿Come en restaurantes de comida rápida? **Koh**-meh ehn rehs-tah-oo-**rahn**-tehs deh koh-**mee**-dah **rah**-pee-dah?

Common Terms for Jaundice

I need to do blood tests.	Necesito hacerle pruebas de sangre. Neh-seh-**see**-toh ah-**sehr**-leh **proo-eh**-bahs deh **sahn**-greh.

I need to do a hepatitis test.

Necesito hacerle una prueba de la hepatitis.
Neh-seh-**see**-toh ah-**sehr**-leh **oo**-nah **proo-eh**-bah deh lah eh-pah-**tee**-tees.

He / she needs an ultrasound of the liver.

Necesita un ultrasonido del hígado.
Neh-seh-**see**-tah oon **ool**-trah-soh-**nee**-doh dehl **ee**-gah-doh.

We need to admit him / her.

Necesitamos internarlo (la).
Neh-seh-see-**tah**-mohs **een**-tehr-**nahr**-loh (lah).

Discharge Instructions for Jaundice

Return to the hospital if he / she has . . .

Regrese al hospital si él / ella tiene . . .
Reh-**greh**-seh ahl **ohs**-pee-tahl see ehl / eh-yah **tee-eh**-neh . . .

___ fever

___ fiebre
fee-eh-breh

___ vomiting

___ vómito
boh-mee-toh

___ worsening abdominal pain

___ peor dolor abdominal
peh-**ohr** doh-**lohr** ab-doh-mee-**nahl**

Neurology

Fall / Head Trauma

Caída / Trauma de la cabeza

Kah-**ee**-dah / Trah-oo-mah deh lah kah-**beh**-sah

Did he / she fall?

¿Se cayó?
Seh kah-**yoh?**

From what height did he / she fall?

¿De qué altura se cayó?
Deh **keh** ahl-**too**-rah seh kah-**yoh?**

Did he / she fall while walking / running?

¿Se cayó mientras caminaba / corria?
Seh kah-**yoh** mee-**ehn**-trahs kah-mee-nah-bah / koh-rhee-ah?

Did he / she fall from . . . ?

¿Se cayó de . . . ?
Seh kah-**yoh** deh . . . ?

___ a chair

___ una silla
oo-nah see-yah

___ a table

___ una mesa
oo-nah meh-sah

___ a bed

___ una cama
oo-nah **kah**-mah

___ a kitchen counter

___ el mostrador de la cocina
ehl mohs-trah-**dohr** deh lah koh-**see**-nah

___ the stairs

___ las escaleras
lahs ehs-kah-**leh**-rahs

Did he / she hit his / her head?

¿Él / ella se pegó en la cabeza?
Ehl / eh-yah seh peh-**goh** ehn lah kah-**beh**-sah?

Did he / she hit . . . ?

¿Él / ella se pegó en . . . ?
Ehl / eh-yah seh peh-**goh** ehn . . . ?

___ the face

___ la cara
lah kah-rah

___ the chest

___ el pecho
ehl **peh**-choh

___ the abdomen

___ el abdomen
ehl ab-**doh**-mehn

___ the back

___ la espalda
lah ehs-**pahl**-dah

___ the leg

___ la pierna
lah **pee-ehr**-nah

___ the arm

___ el brazo
ehl **brah**-soh

Did he / she lose consciousness?

¿Él / ella perdió el conocimiento?
Ehl / eh-yah pehr-dee-**oh** ehl koh-noh-see-mee-**ehn**-toh?

How long did he / she lose consciousness?

¿Por cuánto tiempo perdió el conocimiento?
Pohr **kwahn**-toh **tee-ehm**-poh pehr-dee-**oh** ehl koh-noh-see-mee-**ehn**-toh?

Did he / she vomit since the fall?

¿Ha vomitado desde la caída?
Ah boh-mee-**tah**-doh dehs-deh lah kah-**ee**-dah?

Does he / she have problems with coordination / balance since the fall?

¿Tiene problemas con su coordinación / balance desde la caída?
Tee-eh-neh proh-**bleh**-mahs kohn soo koh-ohr-dee-nah-**see-ohn** / bah-**lahn**-seh dehs-deh lah kah-**ee**-dah?

Is he / she sleeping more than usual?

¿Está durmiendo más de lo usual?
Ehs-**tah** doohr-mee-**ehn**-doh mahs deh loh oo-soo-ahl?

Is he / she irritable?

¿Está irritable?
Ehs-**tah** ee-ree-**tah**-bleh?

Is he / she consolable?

¿Está consolable?
Ehs-**tah** kohn-soh-**lah**-bleh?

Have you noticed any seizure activities / convulsions?

¿Ha notado usted actividades epilépticas / convulsiones?
Ah noh-**tah**-doh oos-**tehd** ahk-tee-bee-**dah**-dehs eh-pee-**lep**-tee-kahs / kohn-bool-**see-oh**-nehs?

Is he / she eating well?

¿Está comiendo bien?
Ehs-**tah** koh-mee-**ehn**-doh bee-ehn?

Has he / she been active (playing) since the fall?

¿Ha estado activo (a) (jugando) desde la caída?
Ah ehs-**tah**-doh ahk-**tee**-boh (ah) (hoo-**gahn**-doh) dehs-deh lah kah-**ee**-dah?

Where does he / she have pain?

¿Dónde tiene dolor?
Dohn-deh **tee-eh**-neh doh-**lohr**?

Can he / she walk?	¿Puede caminar? Pweh-de kah-mee-**nahr**?

Common Terms During the Exam for Head Trauma

I need to examine his / her head.	Necesito examinar su cabeza. Neh-seh-**see**-toh eg-sah-mee-**nahr** soo kah-**beh**-sah
He / she needs X-ray of the . . .	Él / ella necesita radiografía de . . . Ehl / eh-yah neh-seh-**see**-tah **rah**-dee-oh-grah-**fee-ah** deh . . .
He / she needs a CT of the head.	Él / ella necesita una tomografía de la cabeza. Ehl / eh-yah neh-seh-**see**-tah oo-nah toh-moh-grah-**fee-ah** deh lah kah-**beh**-sah.
He / she has a skull fracture.	Él / ella tiene una fractura del cráneo. Ehl / eh-yah **tee-eh**-neh oo-nah frag-**too**-rah dehl **krah**-neh-oh.
He / she has a brain hemorrhage.	Él / ella tiene una hemorragia del cerebro. Ehl / eh-yah **tee-eh**-neh oo-nah eh-moh-**rha**-hee-ah dehl seh-**reh**-broh.
He / she has a brain hematoma.	Él / ella tiene un hematoma del cerebro. Ehl / eh-yah **tee-eh**-neh oon eh-mah-**toh**-mah dehl seh-**reh**-broh.

He / she needs surgery.

Él / ella necesita cirugía (una operación).
Ehl / eh-yah neh-seh-**see**-tah see-roo-**hee**-ah (oo-nah oh-peh-rah-**see-ohn**).

He / she has a bruise.

Él / ella tiene un moretón.
Ehl / eh-yah **tee-eh**-neh oohn moh-reh-**tohn**.

His / her X-rays are fine.

Sus radiografías están bien.
Soos **rah**-dee-oh-grah-**fee-ahs** ehs-**tahn** bee-ehn.

We need to admit him / her.

Necesitamos internarlo (la).
Neh-seh-see-**tah**-mohs **een**-tehr-**nahr**-loh (lah).

Discharge Instructions for Head Trauma

Return to the hospital immediately if the child has . . .

Regrese al hospital inmediatamente si el niño / la niña tiene . . .
Reh-**greh**-seh ahl **ohs**-pee-tahl een-meh-dee-ah-tah-**mehn**-teh see ehl **nee**-nyoh / lah **nee**-nyah **tee-eh**-neh . . .

—— vomiting

—— vómito
boh-mee-toh

—— seizures

—— convulsiones
kohn-bool-**see-oh**-nehs

—— problems with his / her balance / coordination

—— problemas con su balance / coordinación
proh-**bleh**-mahs kohn soo bah-**lahn**-seh / ko-ohr-dee-nah-**see-ohn**

___ headache

___ dolor de cabeza
doh-**lohr** deh kah-**beh**-
sah

___ behavior changes

___ cambio en su
comportamiento
kahm-bee-oh ehn soo
kohm-pohr-tah-mee-**ehn**-
toh

It is okay if he / she wants to
sleep.

Está bien si él / ella quiere
dormir.
Ehs-**tah** bee-ehn see ehl / eh-
yah kee-**eh**-reh dohr-**meer.**

Wake him / her up every two
hours.

Levántelo (la) cada dos horas.
Leh-**bahn**-teh-loh (lah) kah-dah
dohs **oh**-rahs.

Bring him / her back to the
hospital if unable to wake him
/ her up.

Traígalo (la) al hospital si
usted no puede despertarlo
(la).
Trah-ee-gah-loh (lah) ahl ohs-
pee-tahl see oos-**tehd** noh
pweh-deh dehs-pehr-**tahr**-loh
(lah).

Headache

Dolor de Cabeza

Doh-**lohr** deh kah-**beh**-sah

Where does he / she have the
pain?

¿Dónde tiene el dolor?
Dohn-deh **tee-eh**-neh ehl doh-
lohr?

Does he / she have pain in the
forehead?

¿Tiene dolor en la frente?
Tee-eh-neh doh-**lohr** ehn lah
frehn-teh?

Does he / she have pain on the right side of the head?	¿Tiene dolor en el lado derecho de la cabeza? **Tee-eh**-neh doh-**lohr** ehn ehl lah-doh deh-**reh**-choh deh lah kah-**beh**-sah?
Does he / she have pain on the left side of the head?	¿Tiene dolor en el lado izquierdo de la cabeza? **Tee-eh**-neh doh-**lohr** ehn ehl lah-doh ees-**kee-ehr**-doh deh lah kah-**beh**-sah?
Does he / she have pain in the back of the head?	¿Tiene dolor en la parte posterior de la cabeza? **Tee-eh**-neh doh-**lohr** ehn lah pahr-teh pohs-teh-ree-ohr deh lah kah-**beh**-sah?
Does he / she have pain in the nape?	¿Tiene dolor en la nuca? **Tee-eh**-neh doh-**lohr** ehn lah noo-kah?
Does he / she have pain in the neck?	¿Tiene dolor en el cuello? **Tee-eh**-neh doh-**lohr** ehn ehl **kweh**-yoh?
Does he / she have a stiff / rigid neck?	¿Tiene el cuello tieso / rígido? **Tee-eh**-neh ehl **kweh**-yoh **tee-eh**-soh / **ree**-hee-doh?
When did the pain start?	¿Cuándo empezó el dolor? **Kwahn**-doh ehm-peh-**soh** ehl doh-**lohr?**
___ Today	___ Hoy Oy
___ Yesterday	___ Ayer Ah-**yehr**
___ Days	Hace ___ días. Ah-seh **dee**-ahs

Does he / she have fever?	¿Tiene fiebre? **Tee-eh**-neh **fee-eh**-breh?
Does he / she have vomiting?	¿Tiene vómito? **Tee-eh**-neh **boh**-mee-toh?
Does he / she have a sore throat?	¿Tiene dolor de garganta? **Tee-eh**-neh doh-**lohr** deh gahr-**gahn**-tah?
Does he / she have an earache?	¿Tiene dolor de oído? **Tee-eh**-neh doh-**lohr** deh oh-**ee**-doh?
Does he / she have a rash?	¿Tiene manchas / ronchas de la piel? **Tee-eh**-neh **mahn**-chahs / **rhon**-chahs deh lah pee-ehl?
Did he / she receive a blow to the head?	¿Recibió un golpe a la cabeza? Reh-see-bee-**oh** oon **gohl**-peh ah lah kah-**beh**-sah?
Did he / she fall?	¿Se cayó? Seh kah-**yoh?**
What makes the pain worse?	¿Con qué se empeora el dolor? Kohn **keh** seh ehm-peh-**oh**-rah ehl doh-**lohr?**
___ Standing	___ Pararse Pah-**rahr**-seh
___ Lying down	___ Acostarse Ah-kohs-**tahr**-seh
___ The light	___ La luz Lah loos
___ The sun	___ El sol Ehl sohl

What makes the pain better?

¿Con qué se mejora el dolor?
Kohn **keh** seh meh-**ho**-rah ehl doh-**lohr?**

___ Tylenol

___ Tylenol
Tay-leh-nohl

___ Advil

___ Advil
Ahd-beel

___ Eating

___ Comer
Koh-**mehr**

___ Sleeping

___ Dormir
Dohr-**meer**

Did he / she miss school / work because of the headache?

¿Faltó a la escuela / el trabajo por el dolor de cabeza?
Fahl-**toh** ah lah ehs-**kweh**-lah / ehl trah-**bah**-hoh pohr ehl doh-**lohr** deh kah-**beh**-sah?

Does he / she feel numbness on the right side of the body?

¿Siente entumido el lado derecho del cuerpo?
See-ehn-teh ehn-too-**mee**-doh ehl lah-doh deh-**reh**-choh dehl **kwehr**-poh?

Does he / she feel numbness on the left side of the body?

¿Siente entumido el lado izquierdo del cuerpo?
See-ehn-teh ehn-too-**mee**-doh ehl lah-doh ees-**kee-ehr**-doh dehl **kwehr**-poh?

Does he /she have weakness on the right side of the body?

¿Tiene debilidad del lado derecho del cuerpo?
Tee-eh-neh deh-bee-lee-**dahd** dehl lah-doh deh-**reh**-choh dehl **kwehr**-poh?

Does he / she have weakness on the left side of the body?	¿Tiene debilidad del lado izquierdo del cuerpo? **Tee-eh**-neh deh-bee-lee-**dahd** dehl lah-doh ees-**kee-ehr**-doh dehl **kwehr**-poh?

Common Terms During the Exam for Headache

What is your name?	¿Cuál es su nombre? **Kwahl** ehs soo nohm-breh?
How old are you?	¿Cuántos años tiene? **Kwahn**-tohs **ah**-nyohs **tee-eh**-neh?
Do you know where you are?	¿Sabe dónde está? Sah-beh **dohn**-deh ehs-**tah**?
Squeeze my hand hard.	Apriete mi mano fuerte. Ah-**pree-eh**-teh mee **mah**-noh **fwehr**-teh.
Pull me toward you.	Jáleme hacia ti. **Ha**-leh-meh ah-see-ah tee.
Walk a straight line.	Camine una línea derecha. Kah-**mee**-neh oo-nah **lee**-neh-ah deh-**reh**-chah.
Touch your chest with your chin.	Toque su pecho con su mentón. Toh-keh soo **peh**-choh kohn soo mehn-**tohn**.
He / she needs a CT scan of the brain.	Necesita un CT / tomografía del cerebro. Neh-seh-**see**-tah oon seh-teh toh-moh-grah-**fee**-ah dehl seh-**reh**-broh

I need to do a lumbar puncture.	Necesito hacerle una punción lumbar. Neh-seh-**see**-toh ah-**sehr**-leh oo-nah poon-**see-ohn** loom-**bahr.**
He / she has migraines.	Tiene migrañas. **Tee-eh**-neh mee-**grah**-nyahs.
He/she has a viral infection.	Tiene una infección viral. **Tee-eh**-neh oo-nah een-**feg-see**-ohn bee-**rahl.**
He / she has a tumor.	Tiene un tumor. **Tee-eh**-neh oon too-**mohr.**

Discharge Instructions for Headache

Give him / her one tablet of medicine every ___ hours.	Déle una tableta de medicina cada ___ horas. **Deh**-leh oo-nah tah-bleh-tah deh meh-dee-**see**-nah kah-dah ___ **oh**-rahs.
Return to the hospital if he / she has . . .	Regrese al hospital si tiene . . . Reh-**greh**-seh ahl **ohs**-pee-tahl see **tee-eh**-neh . . .
___ vomiting	___ vómito **boh**-mee-toh
___ fever	___ fiebre **fee-eh**-breh
___ worsening headache	___ peor dolor de cabeza peh-**ohr** doh-**lohr** deh kah-**beh**-sah

__ seizures

__ syncope

__ convulsiones
kohn-bool-**see-oh**-nehs

__ desmayo
dehs-**mah**-yoh

Seizures

Convulsiones o Ataques Epilépticos

Kohn-bool-**see-ohn**-ehs oh ah-**tah**-kehs eh-pee-**lep**-tee-kohs

When did the convulsion occur?

¿Cuándo le ocurrió la convulsión?
Kwahn-doh leh oh-koo-**rhee-oh** lah kohn-bool-**see-ohn?**

It has been __ hours.

Hace __ horas.
Ah-seh **oh**-rahs.

__ days

__ días
__ **dee**-ahs

How was the attack?

¿Cómo fué el ataque?
Koh-moh **fweh** ehl ah-**tah**-keh?

__ General seizure

__ Convulsión general
Kohn-bool-**see-ohn** heh-neh-**rahl**

__ Seizure on one side of the body

__ Convulsión en una sola parte del cuerpo
Kohn-bool-**see-ohn** ehn **oo**-nah soh-lah pahr-teh dehl **kwehr**-poh

___ Arm

___ Brazo
Brah-soh

___ Leg

___ Pierna
Pee-ehr-nah

___ Face

___ Cara
Kah-rah

___ Stopped breathing,
turned pale and limp

___ Dejó de respirar, se puso
pálido y sin fuerza
Deh-**hoh** deh rehs-pee-
rahr, seh poo-soh **pah**-
lee-doh ee seen **fwehr**-
sah

___ Stopped breathing,
turned blue and stiff

___ Dejó de respirar, se puso
morado y tieso
Deh-**hoh** deh rehs-pee-
rahr, seh poo-soh moh-
rah-doh ee **tee-eh**-soh

___ Provoked by scolding /
anger / upset

___ Provocado por un
regaño / enojo / disgusto
Proh-boh-**kah**-doh pohr
oon reh-**gah**-nyoh / eh-
noh-ho / dees-**goos**-toh

___ Lost consciousness

___ Perdió el conocimiento
Pehr-**dee-oh** ehl koh-
noh-see-**mee-ehn**-toh

___ Turned stiff (rigid) with
the attack

___ Se puso tieso (rigido)
con el ataque
Seh poo-soh **tee-eh**-soh
(**ree**-hee-doh) kohn ehl
ah-**tah**-keh

___ Turned limp (flaccid)
and weak with the attack

___ Se puso aguado (flácido)
y débil con el ataque
Seh poo-soh ah-**gwah**-
doh (**flah**-see-doh) ee
deh-beel kohn ehl ah-
tah-keh

After the convulsion did he /
she remain asleep or
unconscious?

¿Después de la convulsión
permaneció dormido o
inconciente?
Dehs-**pwehs** deh lah kohn-
bool-**see-ohn** pehr-mah-neh-
see-**oh** dohr-**mee**-doh oh een-
kohn-**see-ehn**-teh?

Did he / she regain
consciousness . . . ?

¿Recobró el
conocimiento . . . ?
Reh-koh-**broh** ehl koh-noh-see-
mee-ehn-toh . . . ?

___ rapidly

___ rápidamente
rah-pee-dah-mehn-teh

___ slowly

___ lentamente
lehn-tah-**mehn**-teh

How long did the convulsion
last?

¿Cuánto tiempo duró la
convulsión?
Kwahn-toh **tee-ehm**-poh doo-
roh lah kohn-bool-**see-ohn?**

___ More than 15 minutes

___ Más de 15 minutos
Mahs deh **keen**-seh
mee-**noo**-tohs

___ Less than 15 minutes

___ Menos de 15 minutos
Meh-nohs deh **keen**-seh
mee-**noo**-tohs

Did he / she have a fever
before the attack or
convulsion?

¿Tenía fiebre antes de darle el
ataque o convulsión?
Teh-**nee**-ah **fee-eh**-breh ahn-
tehs deh dahr-leh ehl ah-**tah**-
keh oh kohn-bool-**see-ohn?**

Has he / she had more than
one attack in 24 hours?

¿Ha tenido más de un ataque
en 24 horas?
Ah teh-**nee**-doh mahs deh oon
ah-**tah**-keh ehn **bein**-tee-**kwah**-
troh **oh**-rahs?

Has he / she ever had attacks like this?

¿Alguna vez ha tenido ataques como este?

Ahl-**goo**-nah behs ah teh-**nee**-doh ah-**tah**-kehs **koh**-moh ehs-teh?

Have they ever told you that he / she has epilepsy?

¿Alguna vez le han dicho que tiene epilepsia?

Ahl-**goo**-nah behs leh ahn dee-choh **keh tee-eh**-neh eh-pee-**lep**-see-ah?

Has he / she hit his / her head recently?

¿Se ha golpeado la cabeza recientemente?

Seh ah gohl-peh-**ah**-doh lah kah-**beh**-sah reh-see-ehn-teh-**mehn**-teh?

Was your baby born premature?

¿Nació su bebé prematuro?

Nah-**see-oh** soo beh-**beh** preh-mah-**too**-roh?

If premature, at how many weeks or months was he / she born?

¿Si fué prematuro, a las cuántas semanas o meses nació?

See **fweh** preh-mah-**too**-roh, ah lahs **kwahn**-tahs seh-**mah**-nahs oh **meh**-sehs nah-**see-oh?**

Does he / she have a problem with the brain?

¿Tiene algún problema con el cerebro?

Tee-eh-neh ahl-**goon** proh-**bleh**-mah kohn ehl seh-**reh**-broh?

Does he / she have a family member with epilepsy?

¿Tiene algún familiar con epilepsia?

Tee-eh-neh ahl-**goon** fah-mee-lee-**ahr** kohn eh-pee-**lep**-see-ah?

___ Baby's mother or father

___ Baby's siblings

Does he / she have a family
member who has seizures
when febrile?

Is the baby taking medication?

Did you notice if he / she
took pills of yours or some
relative?

Does he / she have fever?

Does he / she have a cold or
flu?

Does he / she have vomiting?

___ Padre o madre del bebé
Pah-dreh oh mah-dreh
dehl beh-**beh**

___ Hermanos del bebé
Ehr-**mah**-nohs dehl beh-
beh

¿Tiene algún familiar que le
den ataques cuando tiene
fiebre?
Tee-eh-neh ahl-**goon** fah-mee-
lee-**ahr keh** leh dehn ah-**tah**-
kehs **kwahn**-doh **tee-eh**-neh
fee-eh-breh?

¿Está tomando medicina el
bebé?
Ehs-**tah** toh-**mahn**-doh meh-
dee-**see**-nah ehl beh-**beh?**

¿Se ha dado cuenta si tomó
algunas pastillas de usted o de
algún familiar?
Seh ah dah-doh kwehn-tah
see toh-**moh** ahl-**goo**-nahs
pahs-**tee**-yahs deh oos-**tehd** o
deh ahl-**goon** fah-mee-lee-
ahr?

¿Tiene fiebre?
Tee-eh-neh **fee-eh**-breh?

¿Tiene catarro o gripa?
Tee-eh-neh kah-**tah**-rhoh oh
gree-pah?

¿Tiene vómito?
Tee-eh-neh **boh**-mee-toh?

Does he / she have diarrhea?

¿Tiene diarrea?
Tee-eh-neh dee-ah-**rhe-ah?**

Have you given aspirin or Tylenol?

¿Le ha dado aspirina o Tylenol?
Le ah dah-doh ahs-pee-**ree**-nah oh Tay-leh-nohl?

How many drops or teaspoons?

¿Cuántas gotas o cucharadas?
Kwahn-tahs **goh**-tahs oh koo-cha-**rah**-dahs?

Every how many hours?

¿Cada cuántas horas?
Kah-dah **kwahn**-tahs **oh**-rahs?

Have you rubbed your baby with alcohol?

¿Ha frotado a su bebé con alcohol?
Ah froh-tah-doh ah soo beh-**beh** kohn ahl-**kohl?**

Has he / she been eating well?

¿Ha estado comiendo bien?
Ah ehs-**tah**-doh koh-mee-**ehn**-doh bee-ehn?

Was he / she acting normal before the seizure?

¿Estaba actuando normal antes del ataque?
Ehs-**tah**-bah ahk-too-**ahn**-doh nohr-**mahl ahn**-tehs dehl ah-**tah**-keh?

Was he / she sleeping more than usual before the seizure?

¿Dormía más de lo usual antes del ataque?
Dohr-**mee**-ah mahs deh loh oo-soo-ahl **ahn**-tehs dehl ah-**tah**-keh?

Was he / she more fussy than usual before the seizure?

¿Estaba más molesto de lo usual antes del ataque?
Ehs-**tah**-bah mahs moh-**lehs**-toh deh loh oo-soo-ahl **ahn**-tehs dehl ah-**tah**-keh?

Did you have problems
consoling him / her today?

¿Tuvo problemas al consolarlo
(la) hoy?
Too-boh proh-**bleh**-mahs ahl
kohn-soh-**lahr**-loh (lah) oy?

Common Terms During the Exam for Seizures

Your child has a febrile
seizure.

Su niño (a) tiene convulsiones
de fiebre.
Soo **nee**-nyoh (ah) **tee-eh**-neh
kohn-bool-**see-ohn**-ehs deh
fee-eh-breh.

We need to do blood and
urine analysis.

Necesitamos hacerle análisis
de sangre y orina.
Neh-seh-see-**tah**-mohs ah-
sehr-leh ah-**nah**-lee-sees deh
sahn-greh ee oh-**ree**-nah.

Your child needs an IV.

Su niño (a) necesita suero.
Soo **nee**-nyoh (ah) neh-seh-
see-tah soo-eh-roh.

Your child needs a lumbar
puncture.

Su niño (a) necesita una
punción lumbar.
Soo **nee**-nyoh (ah) neh-seh-
see-tah oo-nah poon-**see-ohn**
loom-**bahr.**

We need to wait for lab
results.

Necesitamos esperar los
resultados de laboratorio.
Neh-seh-see-**tah**-mohs ehs-
peh-**rahr** lohs reh-sool-**tah**-
dohs deh lah-boh-rah-**toh**-ree-
oh.

We need to give him / her
medicine to control the
seizures.

Necesitamos darle medicina
para controlar las
convulsiones.
Neh-seh-see-**tah**-mohs dahr-
leh meh-dee-**see**-nah pah-rah
kohn-troh-**lahr** lahs kohn-bool-
see-oh-nehs.

We need to give him / her antibiotics.

Necesitamos darle antibióticos.
Neh-seh-see-**tah**-mohs dahr-leh ahn-tee-bee-**oh**-tee-kohs.

We need to treat his / her fever.

Necesitamos tratar su fiebre.
Neh-seh-see-**tah**-mohs trah-**tahr** soo **fee-eh**-breh.

Your child needs a CT.

Su niño (a) necesita un CT.
Soo **nee**-nyoh (ah) neh-seh-**see**-tah oon seh-teh.

Your child has (does not have) meningitis.

Su niño (a) tiene (no tiene) meningitis.
Soo **nee**-nyoh (ah) **tee-eh**-neh (noh **tee-eh**-neh) meh-neen-**hee**-tees.

Your child has (does not have) a brain tumor.

Su niño (a) tiene (no tiene) un tumor en el cerebro.
Soo **nee**-nyoh (ah) **tee-eh**-neh (noh **tee-eh**-neh) oon too-**mohr** ehn ehl seh-**reh**-broh.

Discharge Instructions for Seizures

Return to the hospital if the child . . .

Regrese al hospital si el niño (a) . . .
Reh-**greh**-seh ahl **ohs**-pee-tahl see ehl **nee**-nyoh (ah) . . .

___ continues to have seizures

___ continua teniendo ataques epilépticos
kohn-tee-noo-ah teh-nee-**ehn**-doh ah-**tah**-kehs eh-pee-**lep**-tee-kohs

— has trouble walking or talking

— tiene problemas al caminar o hablar
tee-eh-neh proh-**bleh**-mahs ahl kah-mee-**nahr** oh ah-**blahr**

— doesn't have seizure medication

— no tiene medicina para los ataques epilépticos
noh **tee-eh**-neh meh-dee-**see**-nah pah-rah lohs ah **tah** kehs oh pae **lep**-tee-kohs

PART **E**

Orthopedics

Child with a Limp

Niño con Cojera

Nee-nyoh kohn **koh**-he-rah

How long has he had trouble walking?

¿Cuánto tiempo lleva con dificultad al caminar?
Kwahn-toh **tee-ehm**-poh **yeh**-bah kohn dee-fee-kool-**tahd** ahl kah-mee-**nahr?**

It's been ___ hours

___ days

Hace ___ horas
Ah-seh **oh**-rahs

___ días
dee-ahs

Did he / she fall?

¿Se cayó?
Seh kah-**yoh?**

From what height did he / she fall?

¿De qué altura se cayó?
Deh **keh** ahl-**too**-rah seh kah-**yoh?**

___ From the bed

___ De la cama
Deh lah **kah**-mah

___ From the table

___ De la mesa
Deh lah **meh**-sah

___ From a chair

___ De la silla
Deh lah **see**-yah

___ From a bicycle

___ De la bicicleta
Deh lah bee-see-**kleh**-tah

___ While walking

___ Mientras caminaba
Mee-ehn-trahs kah-mee-**nah**-bah

___ While running

___ Mientras corría
Mee-ehn-trahs koh-**ree**-ah

Did he / she hit something?

¿Se pegó contra algo?
Seh peh-**goh kohn**-trah ahl-goh?

Does he / she complain of pain in . . . ?

Se queja de dolor en . . . ?
Seh **keh**-ha deh doh-**lohr** ehn . . . ?

___ the leg

___ la pierna
lah **pee-ehr**-nah

___ the knee

___ la rodilla
lah roh-**dee**-yhah

___ the foot

___ el pie
ehl pee-eh

___ the hip

___ la cadera
lah kah-**deh**-rah

Is it swollen?

¿Está hinchado?
Ehs-**tah** een-**chah**-doh?

Does he / she have bruises?

¿Tiene moretones?
Tee-eh-neh moh-reh-**toh**-nehs?

Is it red or warm?

¿Está rojo o caliente?
Ehs-**tah roh**-ho oh kah-lee-**ehn**-teh?

Does he / she have other joints that are swollen?

¿Tiene otras articulaciones que estén hinchadas?
Tee-eh-neh oh-trahs ahr-tee-koo-lah-**see-oh**-nehs **keh** ehs-**tehn** een-**chah**-dahs?

Does he / she have fever?

¿Tiene fiebre?
Tee-eh-neh **fee-eh** breh?

Does he / she have a cold?

¿Tiene catarro?
Tee-eh-neh kah-**tah**-rho?

Common Terms for Limp

I need to take an X-ray.

Necesito sacarle una radiografía.
Neh-seh-**see**-toh sah-**kahr**-leh **oo**-nah **rah**-dee-oh-grah-**fee-ah.**

I need to do a blood test.

Necesito hacerle una prueba de sangre.
Neh-seh-**see**-toh ah-**sehr**-leh **oo**-nah **proo-eh**-bah deh **sahn**-greh.

I need to do a bone scan.

Necesito hacerle un escán de los huesos.
Neh-seh-**see**-toh ah-**sehr**-leh oon ehs-**kahn** deh lohs **weh**-sohs.

I need to do an ultrasound.

Necesito hacerle un ultrasonido.
Neh-seh-**see**-toh ah-**sehr**-leh oon **ool**-trah-soh-**nee**-doh.

He / she has an infection in the . . .

Él / ella tiene una infección en la . . .
Ehl / eh-yah **tee-eh**-neh **oo**-nah een-feg-**see-ohn** ehn lah . . .

___ hip

___ cadera
kah-**deh**-rah

___ knee

___ rodilla
roh-**dee**-yhah

He / she has a fracture / sprain in . . .

Él / ella tiene una fractura / torcedura en . . .
Ehl / eh-yah **tee-eh**-neh **oo**-nah frag-**too**-rah/tohr-seh-**doo**-rah ehn . . .

___ the hip

___ la cadera
lah kah-**deh**-rah

___ the knee

___ la rodilla
lah roh-**dee**-yhah

___ the leg

___ la pierna
lah **pee-ehr**-nah

___ the ankle

___ el tobillo
ehl toh-**bee**-yhoh

Discharge Instructions for Limp

Give him / her the medicine ___ times a day.

Déle la medicina ___ veces al día.
Deh-leh lah meh-dee-**see**-nah ___ **beh**-sehs ahl **dee**-ah.

Give him / her Tylenol ___ times a day.

Déle Tylenol ___ veces al día.
Deh-leh Tay-leh-nohl ___ **beh**-sehs ahl **dee**-ah.

Return to the hospital if . . .

Regrese al hospital si . . .
Reh-**greh**-seh ahl **ohs**-pee-tahl see . . .

___ he / she has a fever

___ él / ella tiene fiebre
éhl / eh-yah **tee-eh**-neh **fee-eh**-breh

___ the swelling is worse

___ la hinchazón está peor
lah een-chah-**sohn** ehs-**tah** peh-**ohr**

___ he / she has difficulty
walking

___ él / ella tiene dificultad
para caminar
ehl / eh-yah **tee-eh**-neh
dee-fee-kool-**tahd** pah-
rah kah-mee-**nahr**

Ankle Pain / Trauma

Dolor / Trauma de Tobillo

Doh-**lohr** / Trah-oo-mah deh
toh-**bee**-yhoh

When did the pain start?

¿Cuándo empezó el dolor?
Kwahn-doh ehm-peh-**soh** ehl
doh-**lohr?**

___ Today

___ Hoy
Oy

___ Yesterday

___ Ayer
Ah-**yehr**

___ Days ago

Hace ___ días
Ah-seh   **dee**-ahs

Did he / she fall . . . ?

¿Se cayó . . . ?
Seh kah-**yoh** . . . ?

___ while walking

___ mientras caminaba
mee-ehn-trahs kah-mee-
nah-bah

___ while running

___ mientras corria
mee-ehn-trahs koh-**rhee**-
ah

___ while playing sports	___ mientras jugaba deportes **mee-ehn**-trahs hoo-**gah**- bah deh-**pohr**-tehs
___ while skating	___ mientras patinaba **mee-ehn**-trahs pah-tee- **nah**-bah
Did he / she twist the ankle . . . ?	¿Se torció el tobillo . . . ? Seh tohr-**see-oh** ehl toh-**bee**- yohn . . . ?
___ toward the inside	___ hacia adentro **ah**-see-ah ah-**dehn**-troh
___ toward the outside	___ hacia afuera **ah**-see-ah ah-**fweh**-rah
Does he / she have swelling?	¿Tiene hinchazón? **Tee-eh**-neh een-chah-**sohn?**
Has he / she been able to walk since the injury?	¿Ha podido caminar desde que se lastimó? Ah poh-**dee**-doh kah-mee-**nahr** dehs-deh **keh** seh lahs-tee- **moh?**
Does he / she have numbness in the foot / toes?	¿Tiene entumido el pie o los dedos de los pies? **Tee-eh**-neh ehn-too-**mee**-doh ehl pee-eh oh lohs **deh**-dohs deh lohs pee-ehs?
Does he / she have weakness in the foot?	¿Tiene debilidad en el pie? **Tee-eh**-neh deh-bee-lee-**dahd** ehn ehl pee-eh?
Does he / she have redness in the ankle / foot?	¿Tiene el tobillo o el pie rojo? **Tee-eh**-neh ehl toh-**bee**-yoh oh ehl pee-eh **roh**-ho?

Does he / she have fever?

¿Tiene fiebre?
Tee-eh-neh **fee-eh**-breh?

Did he / she take medicine for the pain?

¿Tomó medicina para el dolor?
Toh-**moh** meh-dee-**see**-nah pah-rah ehl doh-**lohr?**

When?

¿Cuándo?
Kwahn-doh?

Common Terms for Ankle Pain

I am going to examine his / her ankle / foot.

Voy a examinar su tobillo / pie.
Boy ah eg-sah-mee-**nahr** soo toh-**bee**-yhoh / pee-eh.

Tell me if it hurts when I touch you here.

Dígame si le duele cuando le toco aquí.
Dee-gah-meh see leh dweh-leh **kwahn**-doh leh toh-koh ah-**kee.**

He / she needs an X-ray.

Necesita una radiografía.
Neh-seh-**see**-tah **oo**-nah **rah**-dee-oh-grah-**fee-ah.**

He / she has a fracture.

Tiene una fractura.
Tee-eh-neh **oo**-nah frag-**too**-rah.

He / she has a sprain.

Tiene una torcedura.
Tee-eh-neh **oo**-nah tohr-seh-**doo**-rah.

He / she has a skin infection.

Tiene una infección de la piel.
Tee-eh-neh **oo**-nah een-feg-**see-ohn** deh lah pee-ehl.

He / she has a contusion.	Tiene una contusión. **Tee-eh**-neh **oo**-nah kohn-too-**see-ohn**.
He / she has a dislocation.	Tiene una luxación. **Tee-eh**-neh **oo**-nah looks-ah-**see-ohn**.
He / she needs a cast (posterior mold).	Necesita yeso. Neh-seh-**see**-tah **yen**-soh.
He / she needs antibiotics.	Necesita antibióticos. Noh sch **see** tah ahn-tee-bee-**oh**-tee-kohs.
He / she needs to see a bone specialist.	Él / ella necesita ver al especialista de los huesos. Ehl / eh-yah neh-seh-**see**-tah behr ahl ehs-**peh-see**-ah-lees-tah deh los **weh**-sohs.
He / she needs surgery (operation).	Él / ella necesita cirugía (operación). Ehl / eh-yah neh-seh-**see**-tah see-roo-**hee**-ah (oh-peh-rah-**see-ohn**).

Discharge Instructions for Ankle Pain

Do not remove the posterior mold.	No se quite el yeso. Noh seh kee-teh ehl **yeh**-soh.
Elevate his / her foot as much as possible.	Eleve su pie lo más qué sea posible. Eh-**leh**-beh soo pee-eh loh mahs **keh** seh-ah poh-**see**-bleh.

Put ice on his / her ankle for twenty minutes every six hours for two days.

Ponga hielo en el tobillo por veinte minutos cada seis horas por dos días.
Pohn-gah **yeh**-loh ehn ehl toh-**bee**-yhoh pohr beh-**een**-teh mee-**noo**-tohs kah-dah says **oh**-rahs pohr dohs **dee**-ahs.

Use the crutches to walk.

Use las muletas para caminar.
Oo-seh lahs moo-**leh**-tahs pah-rah kah-mee-**nahr.**

Do not walk on your foot.

No camine con el pie.
Noh kah-**mee**-neh kohn ehl pee-eh.

See the specialist on ___ at ___ o'clock.

Vaya con el especialista el día ___ a la hora ___ .
Bah-yah kohn ehl ehs-**peh-see**-ah-less-tah ehl **dee**-ah ___ ah lah **oh**-rah ___ .

Give him / her Tylenol or Advil for pain every six hours.

Déle Tylenol o Advil para el dolor cada seis horas.
Deh-leh Tay-leh-nohl oh Ad-beel pah-rah ehl doh-**lohr** kah-dah says **oh**-rahs.

Foot Pain / Trauma

Dolor de Pie / Trauma

Doh-**lohr** deh pee-eh / trah-oo-mah

When did the pain start?

¿Cuándo empezó el dolor?
Kwahn-doh ehm-peh-**soh** ehl doh-**lohr?**

___ Today

___ Hoy
Oy

___ Yesterday

___ Ayer
Ah-**yehr**

___ Days ago

Hace ___ días
Ah-seh **dee**-ahs

Did he / she fall . . . ?

¿Se cayó . . . ?
Seh kah-**yoh** . . . ?

___ while walking

___ mientras caminaba
mee-ehn-trahs kah-mee-
nah-bah

___ while running

___ mientras corría
mee-ehn-trahs koh-**rhee**-
ah

___ while playing sports

___ mientras jugaba deportes
mee-ehn-trahs hoo-**gah**-
bah deh-**pohr**-tehs

___ while skating

___ mientras patinaba
mee-ehn-trahs pah-tee-
nah-bah

Did he / she twist the
foot . . . ?

¿Se torció el pie . . . ?
Seh tohr-**see-oh** ehl pee-
eh . . . ?

___ toward the inside

___ hacia adentro
ah-see-ah ah-**dehn**-troh

___ toward the outside

___ hacia afuera
ah-see-ah ah-**fweh**-rah

Did he / she drop something
on his / her foot?

¿Se le cayó algo encima del
pie?
Seh leh kah-**yoh** ahl-goh ehn-
see-mah dehl pee-eh?

What was it?

¿Qué fué?
Keh fweh?

___ A weight

___ Una pesa
Oo-nah **peh**-sah

___ A drawer

___ Un cajón
Oon kah-**hohn**

___ A book

___ Un libro
Oon lee-broh

Does he / she have swelling?

¿Tiene hinchazón?
Tee-eh-neh een-chah-**sohn?**

Has he / she been able to walk since the injury?

¿Ha podido caminar desde que se lastimó?
Ah poh-**dee**-doh kah-mee-**nahr** dehs-deh **keh** seh lahs-tee-**moh?**

Does he / she have numbness in the foot / toes?

¿Tiene entumido el pie o los dedos de los pies?
Tee-eh-neh ehn-too-**mee**-doh ehl pee-eh oh lohs **deh**-dohs deh lohs pee-ehs?

Does he / she have weakness in the foot?

¿Tiene debilidad en el pie?
Tee-eh-neh deh-bee-lee-**dahd** ehn ehl pee-eh?

Does he / she have redness in the ankle/foot?

¿Tiene el tobillo o el pie rojo?
Tee-eh-neh ehl toh-**bee**-yoh oh ehl pee-eh **roh**-ho?

Does he / she have fever?

¿Tiene fiebre?
Tee-eh-neh **fee-eh**-breh?

Did he / she take medicine for the pain?

¿Tomó medicina para el dolor?
Toh-**moh** meh-dee-**see**-nah pah-rah ehl doh-**lohr?**

When?

¿Cuándo?
Kwahn-doh?

Common Term for Foot Pain

I am going to examine his / her ankle / foot.

Voy a examinar su tobillo / pie.
Boy ah eg-sah-mee-**nahr** soo toh-**bee**-yhoh / pee-eh.

Tell me if it hurts when I touch you here.

Dígame si le duele cuando le toco aquí.
Dee-gah-meh see leh dweh-leh **kwahn**-doh leh toh-koh ah-**kee**.

He / she needs an X-ray.

Necesita una radiografía.
Neh-seh-**see**-tah **oo**-nah **rah**-dee-oh-grah-**fee-ah**.

He / she has a fracture.

Tiene una fractura.
Tee-eh-neh **oo**-nah frag-**too**-rah.

He / she has a sprain.

Tiene una torcedura.
Tee-eh-neh **oo**-nah tohr-seh-**doo**-rah.

He / she has a skin infection.

Tiene una infección de la piel.
Tee-eh-neh **oo**-nah een-feg-**see-ohn** deh lah pee-ehl.

He / she has a contusion.

Tiene una contusión.
Tee-eh-neh **oo**-nah kohn-too-**see-ohn**.

He / she has a dislocation.

Tiene una luxación.
Tee-eh-neh **oo**-nah looks-ah-**see-ohn**.

He / she needs a cast (posterior mold).

Necesita yeso.
Neh-seh-**see**-tah **yeh**-soh.

He / she needs antibiotics.	Necesita antibióticos. Neh-seh-**see**-tah ahn-tee-bee-**oh**-tee-kohs.
He / she needs to see a bone specialist.	Él / ella necesita ver al especialista de los huesos. Ehl / eh-yah neh-seh-**see**-tah behr ahl ehs-**peh**-**see**-ah-lees-tah deh los **weh**-sohs.
He / she needs surgery (operation).	Él / ella necesita cirugía (operación). Ehl / eh-yah neh-seh-**see**-tah see-roo-**hee**-ah. (oh-peh-rah-**see-ohn**).

Discharge Instructions for Foot Pain

Do not remove the posterior mold.	No se quite el yeso. Noh seh kee-teh ehl **yeh**-soh.
Elevate his/her foot as much as possible.	Eleve el pie lo más que sea posible. Eh-**leh**-beh ehl pee-eh loh mahs **keh** seh-ah poh-**see**-bleh.
Put ice on his / her foot for twenty minutes every six hours for two days.	Ponga hielo en el pie por veinte minutos cada seis horas por dos días. **Pohn**-gah **yeh**-loh ehn ehl pee-eh pohr beh-**een**-teh mee-**noo**-tohs kah-dah says **oh**-rahs pohr dohs **dee**-ahs.
Use the crutches to walk.	Use las muletas para caminar. **Oo**-seh lahs moo-**leh**-tahs pah-rah kah-mee-**nahr.**
Do not walk on your foot.	No pise con el pie. Noh **pee**-seh kohn ehl pee-eh.

See the specialist on ___ at ___ o'clock.

Vaya con el especialista el día ___ a la hora ___ .
Bah-ya kohn ehl ehs-**peh-see**-ah-lees-tah ehl **dee**-ah ___ ah lah **oh** rah ___ .

Give him / her Tylenol or Advil for pain every six hours.

Déle Tylenol o Advil para el dolor cada seis horas.
Deh-leh Tay-leh-nohl oh Ad-beel pah-rah ehl doh-**lohr** kah-dah says **on**-rahs.

Knee Pain / Trauma

Dolor de Rodilla / Trauma

Doh-**lohr** deh roh-**dee**-yah / trah-oo-mah

When did the pain start?

¿Cuándo empezó el dolor?
Kwahn-doh ehm-peh-**soh** ehl doh-**lohr?**

___ Today

___ Hoy
Oy

___ Yesterday

___ Ayer
Ah-**yehr**

___ Days ago

Hace ___ días
Ah-seh ___ **dee**-ahs

Did he / she fall . . . ?

¿Se cayó . . . ?
Seh kah-**yoh?**

___ while walking

___ mientras caminaba
mee-ehn-trahs kah-mee-**nah**-bah

— while running

    — mientras corria
    mee-ehn-trahs koh-**rhee**-ah

— while playing sports

    — mientras jugaba deportes
    mee-ehn-trahs hoo-**gah**-bah deh-**pohr**-tehs

— while skating

    — mientras patinaba
    mee-ehn-trahs pah-tee-**nah**-bah

— while skiing

    — mientras esquiaba
    mee-ehn-trahs ehs-kee-**ah**-bah

Did he / she twist the knee?

¿Se torció la rodilla?
Seh tohr-**see-oh** lah roh-**dee**-yah?

Did he / she receive a blow to the knee?

¿Recibió un golpe a la rodilla?
Reh-see-**bee-oh** oon **gohl**-peh ah lah roh-**dee**-yah?

What was it?

¿Qué fué?
Keh fweh?

— A baseball bat

    — Un bate de béisbol
    Oon bah-teh deh **beh**-ees-bohl

— A baseball

    — Bola de béisbol
    Boh-lah deh **beh**-ees-bohl

— A kick

    — Una patada
    Oo-nah pah-**tah**-dah

— Someone's head

    — La cabeza de otra persona
    Lah kah-**beh**-sah deh oh-trah pehr-**soh**-nah

Did he / she drop something on his / her knee?

¿Se le cayó algo encima de la rodilla?
Seh leh kah-**yoh** ahl-goh ehn-**see**-mah deh lah roh-**dee**-yah?

What was it?

¿Qué fué?
Keh fweh?

___ A weight

___ Una pesa
Oo-nah **peh**-sah

___ A drawer

___ Un cajón
Oon kah-**hohn**

___ A book

___ un libro
oon lee-broh

Does he / she have swelling?

¿Tiene hinchazón?
Tee-eh-neh een-chah-**sohn?**

Has he / she been able to walk since the injury?

¿Ha podido caminar desde que se lastimó?
Ah poh-**dee**-doh kah-mee-**nahr** dehs-deh **keh** seh lahs-tee-**moh?**

Does he / she have numbness in the leg?

¿Tiene entumida la pierna?
Tee-eh-neh ehn-too-**mee**-dah lah **pee-ehr**-nah?

Does he / she have weakness in the leg?

¿Tiene debilidad en la pierna?
Tee-eh-neh deh-bee-lee-**dahd** ehn lah **pee-ehr**-nah?

Does he / she have redness in the knee?

¿Tiene la rodilla roja?
Tee-eh-neh lah roh-**dee**-yah **roh**-hah?

Does he / she have fever?

¿Tiene fiebre?
Tee-eh-neh **fee-eh**-breh?

Did he / she take medicine for the pain?	¿Tomó medicina para el dolor? Toh-**moh** meh-dee-**see**-nah pah-rah ehl doh-**lohr?**
When?	Cuándo? **Kwahn**-doh?

Common Terms for Knee Pain

I am going to examine his / her knee.	Voy a examinar su rodilla. Boy ah eg-sah-mee-**nahr** soo roh-**dee**-yah.
Raise up your leg.	Levante su pierna. Leh-**bahn**-teh soo **pee-ehr**-nah.
Tell me if it hurts when I touch you here.	Dígame si le duele cuando le toco aquí. **Dee**-gah-meh see leh dweh-leh **kwahn**-doh leh toh-koh ah-**kee.**
He / she needs an X-ray.	Necesita una radiografía. Neh-seh-**see**-tah **oo**-nah **rah**-dee-oh-grah-**fee-ah.**
He / she has a fracture.	Tiene una fractura. **Tee-eh**-neh **oo**-nah frag-**too**-rah.
He / she has a sprain.	Tiene una torcedura. **Tee-eh**-neh **oo**-nah tohr-seh-**doo**-rah.
He / she has a skin infection.	Tiene una infección de la piel. **Tee-eh**-neh oo-nah een-feg-**see-ohn** deh lah pee-ehl.
He / she has a contusion.	Tiene una contusión. **Tee-eh**-neh **oo**-nah kohn-too-**see-ohn.**

He / she has a dislocation.

Tiene una luxación.
Tee-eh-neh **oo**-nah looks-ah-**see-ohn.**

He / she needs a cast
(posterior mold).

Necesita yeso.
Neh-seh-**see**-tah **yeh**-soh.

He / she needs a knee
immobilizer.

Necesita un inmovilizador de
rodilla.
Neh-seh-**see**-tah oon een-moh-
bee-lee-sah-**dohr** deh roh-**dee**-
yah.

He / she needs antibiotics.

Necesita antibióticos.
Neh-seh-**see**-tah ahn-tee-bee-
oh-tee-kohs.

He / she needs to see a bone
specialist.

Él / ella necesita ver al
especialista de los huesos.
Ehl / eh-yah neh-seh-**see**-tah
behr ahl ehs-**peh-see**-ah-lees-
tah deh los **weh**-sohs.

He / she needs surgery
(operation).

Él / ella necesita cirugía
(operación).
Ehl / eh-yah neh-seh-**see**-tah
see-roo-**hee**-ah (oh-peh-rah-
see-ohn).

Discharge Instructions for Knee Pain

Do not remove the posterior
mold.

No se quite el yeso.
Noh seh kee-teh ehl **yeh**-soh.

Elevate his / her knee as much
as possible.

Eleve la rodilla lo más que sea
posible.
Eh-**leh**-beh lah roh-**dee**-yah loh
mahs **keh** seh-ah poh-**see**-
bleh.

Put ice on his / her knee for twenty minutes every six hours for two days.

Ponga hielo en la rodilla por veinte minutos cada seis horas por dos días.
Pohn-gah **yeh**-loh ehn lah roh-**dee**-yah pohr beh-**een**-teh mee-**noo**-tohs kah-dah says **oh**-rahs pohr dohs **dee**-ahs.

Use the crutches to walk.

Use las muletas para caminar.
Oo-seh lahs moo-**leh**-tahs pah-rah kah-mee-**nahr.**

Do not walk on your leg.

No pise con la pierna.
Noh **pee**-seh kohn lah **pee-ehr**-nah.

See the specialist on ___ at ___ o'clock.

Vaya con el especialista el día ___ a la hora ___ .
Bah-yah kohn ehl ehs-**peh-see**-ah-lees-tah ehl **dee**-ah ___ ah lah **oh**-rah ___ .

Give him / her Tylenol or Advil for pain every ___ hours.

Déle Tylenol o Advil para el dolor cada ___ horas.
Deh-leh Tay-leh-nohl oh Ad-beel pah-rah ehl doh-**lohr** kah-dah ___ **oh**-rahs.

Hip Pain / Trauma

Dolor de Cadera / Trauma

Doh-**lohr** deh kah-**deh**-rah / trah-oo-mah

When did the pain start?

¿Cuándo empezó el dolor?
Kwahn-doh ehm-peh-**soh** ehl doh-**lohr?**

__ Today

__ **Hoy**
Oy

__ Yesterday

__ **Ayer**
Ah-**yehr**

__ Days ago

Hace __ **días**
Ah-seh   **dee**-ahs

Did he / she fall . . . ?

¿**Se cayó . . . ?**
Seh-kah-**yoh** . . . ?

__ while walking

__ **mientras caminaba**
mee-ehn-trahs kah-mee-**nah**-bah

__ while running

__ **mientras corría**
meeh-ehn-trahs koh-**rhee**-ah

__ while playing sports

__ **mientras jugaba deportes**
mee-ehn-trahs hoo-**gah**-bah deh-**pohr**-tehs

__ while skating

__ **mientras patinaba**
mee-ehn-trahs pah-tee-**nah**-bah

__ while skiing

__ **mientras esquiaba**
mee-ehn-trahs ehs-kee-**ah**-bah

Did he / she twist the hip?

¿**Se torció la cadera?**
Seh tohr-**see-oh** lah kah-**deh**-rah?

Did he / she receive a blow to the hip?

¿**Recibió un golpe a la cadera?**
Reh-see-**bee-oh** oon **gohl**-peh ah lah kah-**deh**-rah?

What was it?

¿Qué fué?
Keh fweh?

— A baseball bat

— Un bate de béisbol
Oon bah-teh deh **beh**-ees-bohl

— A baseball

— Bola de béisbol
Boh-lah deh **beh**-ees-bohl

— A kick

— Una patada
Oo-nah pah-**tah**-dah

— Someone's head

— La cabeza de otra persona
Lah kah-**beh**-sah deh oh-trah pehr-**soh**-nah

Does he / she have swelling?

¿Tiene hinchazón?
Tee-eh-neh een-chah-**sohn?**

Has he / she been able to walk since the injury?

¿Ha podido caminar desde que se lastimó?
Ah poh-**dee**-doh kah-mee-**nahr** dehs-deh **keh** seh lahs-tee-**moh?**

Does he / she have numbness in the leg?

¿Tiene entumida la pierna?
Tee-eh-neh ehn-too-**mee**-dah lah **pee-ehr**-nah?

Does he / she have weakness in the leg?

¿Tiene debilidad en la pierna?
Tee-eh-neh deh-bee-lee-**dahd** ehn lah **pee-ehr**-nah?

Does he / she have redness in the hip?

¿Tiene la cadera roja?
Tee-eh-neh lah kah-**deh**-rah **roh**-hah?

Does he / she have a fever?   ¿Tiene fiebre?
Tee-eh-neh **fee-eh**-breh?

Did he / she take medicine for the pain?   ¿Tomó medicina para el dolor?
Toh-**moh** meh-dee-**see**-nah pah-rah ehl doh-**lohr?**

When?   ¿Cuándo?
Kwahn-doh?

Common Terms for Hip Pain

I am going to examine his / her hip.   Voy a examinar su cadera.
Boy ah eg-sah-mee-**nahr** soo kah-**deh**-rah.

Raise up your leg.   Levante su pierna.
Leh-**bahn**-teh soo **pee-ehr**-nah.

Tell me if it hurts when I touch you here.   Dígame si le duele cuando le toco aquí.
Dee-gah-meh see leh dweh-leh **kwahn**-doh leh toh-koh ah-**kee.**

He / she needs an X-ray.   Necesita una radiografía.
Neh-seh-**see**-tah **oo**-nah **rah**-dee-oh-grah-**fee-ah.**

He / she has a fracture.   Tiene una fractura.
Tee-eh-neh **oo**-nah frag-**too**-rah.

He / she has a sprain.   Tiene una torcedura.
Tee-eh-neh **oo**-nah tohr-seh-**doo**-rah.

He / she has a skin infection.

Tiene una infección de la piel.
Tee-eh-neh **oo**-nah een-feg-**see-ohn** deh lah pee-ehl.

He / she has a contusion.

Tiene una contusión.
Tee-eh-neh **oo**-nah kohn-too-**see-ohn.**

He / she has a dislocation.

Tiene una luxación.
Tee-eh-neh **oo**-nah looks-ah-**see-ohn.**

He / she needs antibiotics.

Necesita antibióticos.
Neh-seh-**see**-tah ahn-tee-bee-**oh**-tee-kohs.

He / she needs to see a bone specialist.

Él / ella necesita ver al especialista de los huesos.
Ehl / eh-yah neh-seh-**see**-tah behr ehs-**peh-see**-ah-lees-tah deh los **weh**-sohs.

He / she needs surgery (operation).

Él / ella necesita cirugía (operación).
Ehl / eh-yah neh-seh-**see**-tah see-roo-**hee**-ah (oh-peh-rah-**see-ohn**).

Discharge Instructions for Hip Pain

Put ice on his / her hip for twenty minutes every six hours for two days.

Ponga hielo en la cadera por veinte minutos cada seis horas por dos días.
Pohn-gah **yeh**-loh ehn lah kah-**deh**-rah pohr beh-**een**-teh mee-**noo**-tohs kah-dah says **oh**-rahs pohr dohs **dee**-ahs.

Use the crutches to walk.

Use las muletas para caminar.
Oo-seh lahs moo-**leh**-tahs pah-rah kah-mee-**nahr.**

Do not walk on your leg.

No camine con la pierna.
Noh kah-**mee**-neh kohn lah
pee-ehr-nah.

See the specialist on ___ at
___ o'clock.

Vaya con el especialista el día
___ a la hora ___ .
Bah-yah kohn ehl ehs-**peh-
see**-ah-lees-tah ehl **dee**-ah
___ ah lah **oh**-rah ___ .

Give him / her Tylenol or
Advil for pain every ___
hours.

Dele Tylenol o Advil para el
dolor cada ___ horas.
Deh-leh Tay-leh-nohl oh Ad-
beel pah-rah ehl doh-**lohr** kah-
dah ___ **oh**-rahs.

Leg Pain / Trauma

Dolor de Pierna / Trauma

Doh-**lohr** deh **pee-ehr**-nah /
trah-oo-mah

When did the pain start?

¿Cuándo empezó el dolor?
Kwahn-doh ehm-peh-**soh** ehl
doh-**lohr?**

___ Today

___ Hoy
Oy

___ Yesterday

___ Ayer
Ah-**yehr**

___ Days ago

Hace ___ días
Ah-seh **dee**-ahs

Did he / she fall . . . ?

¿Se cayó . . . ?
Seh kah-**yoh** . . . ?

___ while walking

___ mientras caminaba
mee-ehn-trahs kah-mee-**nah**-bah

___ while running

___ mientras corria
mee-ehn-trahs koh-**rhee**-ah

___ while playing sports

___ mientras jugaba deportes
mee-ehn-trahs hoo-**gah**-bah deh-**pohr**-tehs

___ while skating

___ mientras patinaba
mee-ehn-trahs pah-tee-**nah**-bah

___ while skiing

___ mientras esquiaba
mee-ehn-trahs ehs-kee-**ah**-bah

Did he / she twist the leg?

¿Se torció la pierna?
Seh tohr-**see-oh** lah **pee-ehr**-nah?

Did he / she receive a blow to the leg?

¿Recibió un golpe a la pierna?
Reh-see-**bee-oh** oon **gohl**-peh ah lah **pee-ehr**-nah?

What was it?

¿Qué fué?
Keh fweh?

___ A baseball bat

___ Un bate de béisbol
Oon bah-teh deh **beh**-ees-bohl

___ A baseball

___ Una bola de béisbol
Oo-nah boh-lah deh **beh**-ees-bohl

___ A kick

___ Una patada
Oo-nah pah-**tah**-dah

___ Someone's head

___ La cabeza de otra persona
Lah kah-**beh**-sah deh
oh-trah pehr-**soh**-nah

Did he / she drop something on his / her leg?

¿Se le cayó algo encima de la pierna?
Seh leh kah-**yoh** ahl-goh ehn-**see**-mah deh lah **pee-ehr**-nah?

What was it?

¿Qué fué?
Keh fewh?

___ A weight

___ Una pesa
Oo-nah **peh**-sah

___ A drawer

___ Un cajón
Oon kah-**hohn**

___ A book

___ Un libro
Oon lee-broh

Does he / she have swelling?

¿Tiene hinchazón?
Tee-eh-neh een-chah-**sohn?**

Has he / she been able to walk since the injury?

¿Ha podido caminar desde que se lastimó?
Ah poh-**dee** doh kah-mee-**nahr** dehs-deh **keh** seh lahs-tee-**moh?**

Does he / she have numbness in the leg?

¿Tiene entumida la pierna?
Tee-eh-neh ehn-too-**mee**-dah lah **pee-ehr**-nah?

Does he / she have weakness in the leg?

¿Tiene debilidad en la pierna?
Tee-eh-neh deh-bee-lee-**dahd** ehn lah **pee-ehr**-nah?

Does he / she have redness in the leg?	¿Tiene la pierna roja? **Tee-eh**-neh lah **pee-ehr**-nah **roh**-hah?
Does he / she have fever?	¿Tiene fiebre? **Tee-eh**-neh **fee-eh**-breh?
Did he / she take medicine for the pain?	¿Tomó medicina para el dolor? Toh-**moh** meh-dee-**see**-nah pah-rah ehl doh-**lohr?**
When?	¿Cuándo? **Kwahn**-doh?

Common Terms for Leg Pain

I am going to examine his / her leg.	Voy a examinar su pierna. Boh-ee ah eg-sah-mee-**nahr** soo **pee-ehr**-nah.
Raise up your leg.	Levante su pierna. Leh-**bahn**-teh soo **pee-ehr**-nah.
Tell me if it hurts when I touch you here.	Dígame si le duele cuando le toco aquí. **Dee**-gah-meh see leh dweh-leh **kwahn**-doh leh toh-koh ah-**kee.**
He / she needs an X-ray.	Necesita una radiografía. Neh-seh-**see**-tah **oo**-nah **rah**-dee-oh-grah-**fee-ah.**
He / she has a fracture.	Tiene una fractura. **Tee-eh**-neh **oo**-nah frag-**too**-rah.

He / she has a sprain.

Tiene una torcedura.
Tee-eh-neh **oo**-nah tohr-seh-**doo**-rah.

He / she has a skin infection.

Tiene una infección de la piel.
Tee-eh-neh **oo**-nah een-feg-**see-ohn** deh lah pee-ehl.

He / she has a contusion.

Tiene una contusión.
Tee-eh-neh **oo**-nah kohn-too-**see-ohn.**

He / she needs a knee immobilizer.

Necesita un inmovilizador de rodilla.
Neh-seh-**see**-tah oon een-moh-bee-lee-sah-**dohr** deh roh-**dee**-yah.

He / she needs antibiotics.

Necesita antibióticos.
Neh-seh-**see**-tah ahn-tee-bee-**oh**-tee-kohs.

He / she needs to see a bone specialist.

Él / ella necesita ver al especialista de los huesos.
Ehl / eh-yah neh-seh-**see**-tah behr ahl ehs-**peh-see**-ah-lees-tah deh los **weh**-sohs.

He / she needs surgery (operation).

Él / ella necesita cirugía (operación).
Ehl / eh-yah neh-seh-**see**-tah see-roo-**hee**-ah (oh-peh-rah-**see-ohn**).

Discharge Instructions for Leg Pain

Rest your leg as much as possible.

Descanse su pierna lo más que sea posible.
Dehs-**kahn**-seh soo **pee-ehr**-nah loh mahs **keh** seh-ah poh-**see**-bleh.

Put ice on his / her leg for twenty minutes every six hours for two days.

Ponga hielo en la pierna por veinte minutos cada seis horas por dos días.
Pohn-gah **yeh**-loh ehn lah **pee-ehr**-nah pohr beh-**een**-teh mee-**noo**-tohs kah-dah says **oh**-rahs pohr dohs **dee**-ahs.

Use the crutches to walk.

Use las muletas para caminar.
Oo-seh lahs moo-**leh**-tahs pah-rah kah-mee-**nahr.**

Do not walk on the leg.

No camine con la pierna.
Noh kah-**mee**-neh kohn lah **pee-ehr**-nah.

See the specialist on ___ at ___ o'clock.

Vaya con el especialista el día ___ a la hora ___ .
Bah-yah kohn ehl ehs-**peh-see**-ah-lees-tah ehl **dee**-ah ___ ah lah **oh**-rah ___ .

Give him / her Tylenol or Advil for pain every ___ hours.

Déle Tylenol o Advil para el dolor cada ___ horas.
Deh-leh Tay-leh-nohl oh Ad-beel pah-rah ehl doh-**lohr** kah-dah ___ **oh**-rahs.

Hand Pain / Trauma

Dolor de Mano / Trauma

Doh-**lohr** deh **mah**-noh / trah-oo-mah

When did the pain start?

¿Cuándo empezó el dolor?
Kwahn-doh ehm-peh-**soh** ehl doh-**lohr?**

— Today

— Hoy
Oy

— Yesterday

— Ayer
Ah-**yehr**

— Days ago

Hace — días
Ah-seh **dee**-ahs

Did he / she fall . . . ?

¿Se cayó . . . ?
Seh kah **yoh** . . . ?

— while walking

— mientras caminaba
mee-ehn-trahs kah-mee-
nah-bah

— while running

— mientras corria
mee-ehn-trahs koh-**rhee**-
ah

— while playing sports

— mientras jugaba deportes
mee-ehn-trahs hoo-**gah**-
bah deh-**pohr**-tehs

— while skating

— mientras patinaba
mee-ehn-trahs pah-tee-
nah-bah

Did he / she twist the hand?

¿Se torció la mano?
Seh tohr-**see-oh** lah **mah**-noh?

Did he / she drop something
on his / her hand?

¿Se le cayó algo encima de la
mano?
Seh leh kah-**yoh** ahl-goh ehn-
see-mah deh lah **mah**-noh?

What was it?

¿Qué fué?
Keh fweh?

— A weight

— Una pesa
Oo-nah **peh**-sah

___ A drawer

___ Un cajón
Oon kah-**hohn**

___ A book

___ Un libro
Oon lee-broh

Does he / she have swelling?

¿Tiene hinchazón?
Tee-eh-neh een-chah-**sohn?**

Does he / she have numbness
in the fingers?

¿Tiene entumidos los dedos?
Tee-eh-neh ehn-too-**mee**-dohs
lohs **deh**-dohs?

Does he / she have weakness
in the hand?

¿Tiene debilidad en la mano?
Tee-eh-neh deh-bee-lee-**dahd**
ehn lah **mah**-noh?

Does he / she have redness in
the hand?

¿Tiene la mano roja?
Tee-eh-neh lah **mah**-noh **roh**-
hah?

Does he / she have a fever?

¿Tiene fiebre?
Tee-eh-neh **fee-eh**-breh?

Did he / she take medicine for
the pain?

¿Tomó medicina para el
dolor?
Toh-**moh** meh-dee-**see**-nah
pah-rah ehl doh-**lohr?**

When?

¿Cuándo?
Kwahn-doh?

Common Terms for Hand Pain

I am going to examine his /
her hand.

Voy a examinar su mano.
Boy ah eg-sah-mee-**nahr** soo
mah-noh.

Tell me if it hurts when I touch you here.

Dígame si le duele cuándo le toco aquí.
Dee-gah-meh see leh dweh-leh **kwahn**-doh leh toh-koh ah-**kee.**

He / she needs an X-ray.

Necesita una radiografía.
Neh-seh-**see**-tah **oo**-nah **rah**-dee-oh-grah-**fee-ah.**

He / she has a fracture.

Tiene una fractura.
Tee-eh-neh **oo**-nah frag-**too**-rah.

He / she has a sprain.

Tiene una torcedura.
Tee-eh-neh **oo**-nah tohr-seh-**doo**-rah.

He / she has a skin infection.

Tiene una infección de la piel.
Tee-eh-neh **oo**-nah een-feg-**see-ohn** deh lah pee-ehl.

He / she has a contusion.

Tiene una contusión.
Tee-eh-neh **oo**-nah kohn-too-**see-ohn.**

He / she has a dislocation.

Tiene una luxación.
Tee-eh-neh **oo**-nah looks-ah-**see-ohn.**

He / she needs a cast (posterior mold).

Necesita yeso.
Neh-seh-**see**-tah **yeh**-soh.

He / she needs antibiotics.

Necesita antibióticos.
Neh-seh-**see**-tah ahn-tee-bee-**oh**-tee-kohs.

He / she needs to see a bone specialist.

Él / ella necesita ver al especialista de los huesos.
Ehl / eh-yah neh-seh-**see**-tah behr ahl ehs-**peh-see**-ah-lees-tah deh los **weh**-sohs.

He / she needs surgery
(operation).

Él / ella necesita cirugía
(operación).
Ehl / eh-yah neh-seh-**see**-tah
see-roo-**hee**-ah (oh-peh-rah-
see-ohn).

Discharge Instructions for Hand Pain

Do not remove the posterior
mold.

No se quite el yeso.
Noh seh kee-teh ehl **yeh**-soh.

Elevate his / her hand as
much as possible.

Eleve la mano lo más que sea
posible.
Eh-**leh**-beh lah **mah**-noh loh
mahs **keh** seh-ah poh-**see**-
bleh.

Put ice on his / her hand for
twenty minutes every six hours
for two days.

Ponga hielo en la mano por
veinte minutos cada seis horas
por dos días.
Pohn-gah **yeh**-loh ehn lah
mah-noh pohr beh-**een**-teh
mee-**noo**-tohs kah-dah says
oh-rahs pohr dohs **dee**-ahs.

See the specialist on ___ at
___ o'clock.

Vaya con el especialista el día
___ a la hora ___ .
Bah-yah kohn ehl ehs-**peh-
see**-ah-lees-tah ehl **dee**-ah
___ ah lah **oh**-rah ___ .

Give him / her Tylenol or
Advil for pain every ___
hours.

Déle Tylenol o Advil para el
dolor cada ___ horas.
Deh-leh Tay-leh-nohl oh Ad-
beel pah-rah ehl doh-**lohr** kah-
dah ___ **oh**-rahs.

Finger Pain / Trauma

Dolor de Dedo / Trauma

Doh-**lohr** deh **deh**-doh / trah-oo-mah

When did the pain start?

¿Cuándo empezó el dolor?
Kwahn-doh ehm-peh-**soh** ehl doh-**lohr?**

___ Today

___ Hoy
Oy

___ Yesterday

___ Ayer
Ah-**yehr**

___ Days ago

Hace ___ días
Ah-seh   **dee**-ahs

Did he / she fall . . . ?

¿Se cayó . . . ?
Seh kah-**yoh** . . . ?

___ while walking

___ mientras caminaba
mee-ehn-trahs kah-mee-**nah**-bah

___ while running

___ mientras corria
mee-ehn-trahs koh-**rhee**-ah

___ while playing sports

___ mientras jugaba deportes
mee-ehn-trahs hoo-**gah**-bah deh-**pohr**-tehs

___ while skating

___ mientras patinaba
mee-ehn-trahs pah-tee-**nah**-bah

Did he / she twist the finger?

¿Se torció el dedo?
Seh tohr-**see-oh** ehl **deh**-doh?

Did he / she drop something on his/her finger?

¿Se le cayó algo encima del dedo?
Seh leh kah-**yoh** ahl-goh ehn-**see**-mah dehl **deh**-doh?

What was it?

¿Qué fué?
Keh fweh?

___ A weight

___ Una pesa
Oo-nah **peh**-sah

___ A drawer

___ Un cajón
Oon kah-**hohn**

___ A book

___ Un libro
Oon lee-broh

Does he / she have swelling?

¿Tiene hinchazón?
Tee-eh-neh een-chah-**sohn?**

Does he / she have numbness in the finger?

¿Tiene entumido el dedo?
Tee-eh-neh ehn-too-**mee**-doh ehl **deh**-doh?

Does he / she have weakness in the finger?

¿Tiene debilidad en el dedo?
Tee-eh-neh deh-bee-lee-**dahd** ehn el **deh**-doh?

Does he / she have redness in the finger?

¿Tiene el dedo rojo?
Tee-eh-neh ehl **deh**-doh **roh**-ho?

Does he /she have fever?

¿Tiene fiebre?
Tee-eh-neh **fee-eh**-breh?

Did he / she take medicine for the pain?

¿Tomó medicina para el dolor?
Toh-**moh** meh-dee-**see**-nah pah-rah ehl doh-**lohr?**

When?

¿Cuándo?
Kwahn-doh?

Common Terms for Finger Pain

I am going to examine your finger.	Voy a examinar su dedo. Boy ah eg-sah-mee-**nahr** soo **deh**-doh.
Tell me if it hurts when I touch you here.	Dígame si le duele cuando le toco aquí. **Dee**-gah-meh see leh dweh-leh **kwahn**-doh leh toh-koh ah-**kee**.
He / she needs an X-ray.	Necesita una radiografía. Neh-seh-**see**-tah **oo**-nah **rah**-dee-oh-grah-**fee-ah.**
He / she has a fracture.	Tiene una fractura. **Tee-eh**-neh **oo**-nah frag-**too**-rah.
He / she has a sprain.	Tiene una torcedura. **Tee-eh**-neh **oo**-nah tohr-seh-**doo**-rah.
He / she has a skin infection.	Tiene una infección de la piel. **Tee-eh**-neh **oo**-nah een-feg-**see-ohn** deh lah pee-ehl.
He / she has a contusion.	Tiene una contusión. **Tee-eh**-neh **oo**-nah kohn-too-**see-ohn.**
He / she has a dislocation.	Tiene una luxación. **Tee-eh**-neh **oo**-nah looks-ah-**see-ohn.**
He / she needs a splint.	Necesita una férula / tablilla. Neh-seh-**see**-tah oo-**nah feh**-roo-lah / tah-**blee**-yah.
He / she needs antibiotics.	Necesita antibióticos. Neh-seh-**see**-tah ahn-tee-bee-**oh**-tee-kohs.

He / she needs to see a bone specialist.

Él / ella necesita ver al especialista de los huesos.
Ehl / eh-yah neh-seh-**see**-tah behr ahl ehs-**peh-see**-ah-lees-tah deh los **weh**-sohs.

He / she needs surgery (operation).

Él / ella necesita cirugía (operación).
Ehl / eh-yah neh-seh-**see**-tah see-roo-**hee**-ah (oh-peh-rah-**see-ohn**).

Discharge Instructions for Finger / Thumb Pain

Do not remove the splint.

No se quite la férula / tablilla.
Noh seh kee-teh lah **feh**-roo-lah / tah-**blee**-yah.

Elevate his / her hand as much as possible.

Eleve su mano lo más que sea posible.
Eh-**leh**-beh soo **mah**-noh loh mahs **keh** seh-ah poh-**see**-bleh.

Put ice on his / her finger for twenty minutes every six hours for two days.

Ponga hielo en su dedo por veinte minutos cada seis horas por dos días.
Pohn-gah **yeh**-loh ehn soo **deh**-doh pohr beh-**een**-teh mee-**noo**-tohs kah-dah says **oh**-rahs pohr dohs **dee**-ahs.

See the specialist on __ at __ o'clock.

Vaya con el especialista el día __ a la hora __ .
Bah-yah kohn ehl ehs-**peh-see**-ah-lees-tah ehl **dee**-ah __ ah lah **oh**-rah __ .

Give him / her Tylenol or Advil for pain every ___ hours.	Déle Tylenol o Advil para el dolor cada ___ horas. **Deh**-leh Tay-leh-nohl oh Ad-beel pah-rah ehl doh-**lohr** kah-dah ___ **oh**-rahs.

Arm Pain / Trauma

Dolor de Brazo / Trauma

Doh-**lohr** deh **brah**-soh / trah-oo-mah

When did the pain start?	¿Cuándo empezó el dolor? **Kwahn**-doh ehm-peh-**soh** ehl doh-**lohr?**
___ Today	___ Hoy Oy
___ Yesterday	___ Ayer Ah-**yehr**
___ Days ago	Hace ___ días Ah-seh **dee**-ahs
Did he / she fall . . . ?	¿Se cayó . . . ? Seh kah-**yoh** . . . ?
___ while walking	___ mientras caminaba **mee-ehn**-trahs kah-mee-**nah**-bah
___ while running	___ mientras corría **mee-ehn**-trahs koh-**rhee**-ah

—— while playing sports

—— mientras jugaba deportes
mee-ehn-trahs hoo-**gah**-
bah deh-**pohr**-tehs

—— while skating

—— mientras patinaba
mee-ehn-trahs pah-tee-
nah-bah

Did he / she twist the arm?

¿Se torció el brazo?
Seh tohr-**see-oh** ehl **brah**-soh?

Did he / she drop something
on his / her arm?

¿Se le cayó algo encima del
brazo?
Seh leh kah-**yoh** ahl-goh ehn-
see-mah dehl **brah**-soh?

What was it?

¿Qué fué?
Keh fweh?

—— A weight

—— Una pesa
Oo-nah **peh**-sah

—— A drawer

—— Un cajón
Oon kah-**hohn**

—— A book

—— Un libro
Oon lee-broh

Does he / she have swelling?

¿Tiene hinchazón?
Tee-eh-neh een-chah-**sohn?**

Does he / she have numbness
in the arm / hand?

¿Tiene entumido el brazo / la
mano?
Tee-eh-neh ehn-too-**mee**-doh
ehl **brah**-soh / lah **mah**-noh?

Does he / she have weakness
in the arm / hand?

¿Tiene debilidad en el brazo /
la mano?
Tee-eh-neh deh-bee-lee-**dahd**
ehn ehl **brah**-soh / lah **mah**-
noh?

Does he / she have redness in the arm?

¿Tiene el brazo rojo?
Tee-eh-neh ehl **brah**-soh **roh**-ho?

Does he / she have fever?

¿Tiene fiebre?
Tee-eh-neh **fee-eh**-breh?

Did he / she take medicine for the pain?

¿Tomó medicina para el dolor?
Toh-**moh** meh-dee-**see**-nah pah-rah ehl doh-**lohr?**

When?

¿Cuándo?
Kwahn-doh?

Common Terms for Arm Pain

I am going to examine his / her arm.

Voy a examinar su brazo.
Boy ah eg-sah-mee-**nahr** soo **brah**-soh.

Tell me if it hurts when I touch you here.

Dígame si le duele cuando le toco aquí.
Dee-gah-meh see leh dweh-leh **kwahn**-doh leh toh-koh ah-**kee.**

He / she needs an X-ray.

Necesita una radiografía.
Neh-seh-**see**-tah **oo**-nah **rah**-dee-oh-grah-**fee-ah.**

He / she has a fracture.

Tiene una fractura.
Tee-eh-neh **oo**-nah frag-**too**-rah.

He / she has a sprain.

Tiene una torcedura.
Tee-eh-neh **oo**-nah tohr-seh-**doo**-rah.

He / she has a skin infection.

Tiene una infección de la piel.
Tee-eh-neh **oo**-nah een-feg-**see-ohn** deh lah pee-ehl.

He / she has a contusion.

Tiene una contusión.
Tee-eh-neh **oo**-nah kohn-too-**see-ohn.**

He / she has a dislocation.

Tiene una luxación.
Tee-eh-neh **oo**-nah looks-ah-**see-ohn.**

He / she needs a cast (posterior mold).

Necesita yeso.
Neh-seh-**see**-tah **yeh**-soh.

He / she needs antibiotics.

Necesita antibióticos.
Neh-seh-**see**-tah ahn-tee-bee-**oh**-tee-kohs.

He / she needs to see a bone specialist.

Él / ella necesita ver al especialista de los huesos.
Ehl / eh-yah neh-seh-**see**-tah behr ahl ehs-**peh-see**-ah-lees-tah deh los **weh**-sohs.

He / she needs surgery (operation).

Él / ella necesita cirugía (operación).
Ehl / eh-yah neh-seh-**see**-tah see-roo-**hee**-ah (oh-peh-rah-**see-ohn**).

Discharge Instructions for Arm Pain

Do not remove the posterior mold.

No se quite el yeso.
Noh seh kee-teh ehl **yeh**-soh.

Elevate his / her arm as much as possible.

Eleve su brazo lo más que sea posible.
Eh-**leh**-beh soo **brah**-soh loh mahs **keh** seh-ah poh-**see**-bleh.

Put ice on his / her arm for twenty minutes every six hours for two days.

Ponga hielo en su brazo por veinte minutos cada seis horas por dos días.
Pohn-gah **yeh**-loh ehn soo **brah**-soh pohr beh-**een**-teh mee-**noo**-tohs kah-dah says **oh**-rahs pohr dohs **dee**-ahs.

See the specialist on ___ at ___ o'clock.

Vaya con el especialista el día ___ a la hora ___ .
Bah-yah kohn ehl ehs-**peh-see**-ah-lees-tah ehl **dee**-ah ___ ah lah **oh**-rah ___ .

Give him / her Tylenol or Advil for pain every ___ hours.

Déle Tylenol o Advil para el dolor cada ___ horas.
Deh-leh Tay-leh-nohl oh Ad-beel pah-rah ehl doh-**lohr** kah-dah ___ **oh**-rahs.

Wrist Pain / Trauma

Dolor de Muñeca / Trauma

Doh-**lohr** deh moo-**nyeh**-kah / trah-oo-mah

When did the pain start?

¿Cuándo empezó el dolor?
Kwahn-doh ehm-peh-**soh** ehl doh-**lohr?**

___ Today

___ Hoy
Oy

___ Yesterday

___ Ayer
Ah-**yehr**

___ Days ago

Hace ___ días
Ah-seh **dee**-ahs

Did he / she fall . . . ?

¿Se cayó . . . ?
Seh kah-**yoh** . . . ?

___ while walking

___ mientras caminaba
mee-ehn-trahs kah-mee-**nah**-bah

___ while running

___ mientras corria
mee-ehn-trahs koh-**rhee**-ah

___ while playing sports

___ mientras jugaba deportes
mee-ehn-trahs hoo-**gah**-bah deh-**pohr**-tehs

___ while skating

___ mientras patinaba
mee-ehn-trahs pah-tee-**nah**-bah

Did he / she twist the hand / wrist?

¿Se torció la mano / muñeca?
Seh tohr-**see-oh** lah **mah**-noh / lah moo-**nyeh**-kah?

Did he / she drop something on his/her hand / wrist?

¿Se le cayó algo encima de la mano / muñeca?
Seh leh kah-**yoh** ahl-goh ehn-**see**-mah deh lah **mah**-noh / lah moo-**nyeh**-kah?

What was it?

¿Qué fué?
Keh fweh?

___ A weight

___ Una pesa
Oo-nah **peh**-sah

___ A drawer

___ Un cajón
Oon kah-**hohn**

___ A book

___ Un libro
Oon lee-broh

Does he / she have swelling?	¿Tiene hinchazón? **Tee-eh**-neh een-chah-**sohn?**
Does he / she have numbness in the hand / fingers?	¿Tiene entumida (os) la mano / los dedos? **Tee-eh**-neh ehn too-**mee**-dah (ohs) lah **mah**-noh / lohs **deh**-dohs?
Does he / she have weakness in the hand?	¿Tiene debilidad en la mano? **Tee-eh**-neh deh-bee-loo-**dahd** ehn lah **mah**-noh?
Does he / she have redness in the hand / fingers?	¿Tiene la mano / los dedos rojos? **Tee-eh**-neh lah **mah**-noh / lohs **deh**-dohs **roh**-hos?
Does he / she have fever?	¿Tiene fiebre? **Tee-eh**-neh **fee-eh**-breh?
Did he / she take medicine for the pain?	¿Tomó medicina para el dolor? Toh-**moh** meh-dee-**see**-nah pah-rah ehl doh-**lohr?**
When?	¿Cuándo? **Kwahn**-doh?

Common Terms for Wrist Pain

I am going to examine his / her wrist.	Voy a examinar su muñeca. Boy ah eg-sah-mee-**nahr** soo moo-**nyeh**-kah.
Tell me if it hurts when I touch you here.	Dígame si le duele cuando le toco aquí. **Dee**-gah-meh see leh dweh-leh **kwahn**-doh leh toh-koh ah-**kee.**

He / she needs an X-ray.

Necesita una radiografía.
Neh-seh-**see**-tah oo-nah **rah**-dee-oh-grah-**fee-ah.**

He / she has a fracture.

Tiene una fractura.
Tee-eh-neh **oo**-nah frag-**too**-rah.

He / she has a sprain.

Tiene una torcedura.
Tee-eh-neh **oo**-nah tohr-seh-**doo**-rah.

He / she has a skin infection.

Tiene una infección de la piel.
Tee-eh-neh **oo**-nah een-feg-**see-ohn** deh lah pee-ehl.

He / she has a contusion.

Tiene una contusión.
Tee-eh-neh **oo**-nah kohn-too-**see-ohn.**

He / she has a dislocation.

Tiene una luxación.
Tee-eh-neh **oo**-nah looks-ah-**see-ohn.**

He / she needs a cast
(posterior mold).

Necesita yeso.
Neh-seh-**see**-tah **yeh**-soh.

He / she needs antibiotics.

Necesita antibióticos.
Neh-seh-**see**-tah ahn-tee-bee-**oh**-tee-kohs.

He / she needs to see a bone
specialist.

Él / ella necesita ver al
especialista de los huesos.
Ehl / eh-yah neh-seh-**see**-tah behr ahl ehs-**peh-see**-ah-lees-tah deh los **weh**-sohs.

He / she needs surgery
(operation).

Él / ella necesita cirugía
(operación).
Ehl / eh-yah neh-seh-**see**-tah
see-roo-**hee**-ah (oh-peh-rah-
see-ohn.)

Discharge Instructions for Wrist Pain

Do not remove the posterior
mold.

No se quite el yeso.
Noh seh kee-teh ehl **yeh**-soh.

Elevate his / her hand as
much as possible.

Eleve su mano lo más que sea
posible.
Eh-**leh**-beh soo **mah**-noh loh
mahs **keh** seh-ah poh-**see**-
bleh.

Put ice on his / her wrist for
twenty minutes every six hours
for two days.

Ponga hielo en su muñeca por
veinte minutos cada seis horas
por dos días.
Pohn-gah **yeh**-loh ehn soo
moo-**nyeh**-kah pohr beh-**een**-
teh mee-**noo**-tohs kah-dah
says **oh**-rahs pohr dohs **dee**-
ahs.

See the specialist on ___ at
___ o'clock.

Vaya con el especialista el día
___ a la hora ___ .
Bah-yah kohn ehl ehs-**peh**-
see-ah-lees-tah ehl **dee**-ah
___ ah lah **oh**-rah ___ .

Give him / her Tylenol or
Advil for pain every ___
hours.

Déle Tylenol o Advil para el
dolor cada ___ horas.
Deh-leh Tay-leh-nohl oh Ad-
beel pah-rah ehl doh-**lohr** kah-
dah ___ **oh**-rahs.

Elbow Pain / Trauma

Dolor de Codo / Trauma

Doh-**lohr** deh **koh**-doh / trah-oo-mah

When did the pain start?

¿Cuándo empezó el dolor?
Kwahn-doh ehm-peh-**soh** ehl doh-**lohr?**

—— Today

—— Hoy
Oy

—— Yesterday

—— Ayer
Ah-**yehr**

—— Days ago

Hace —— días
Ah-seh   **dee**-ahs

Did he /she fall . . . ?

¿Se cayó . . . ?
Seh kah-**yoh** . . . ?

—— while walking

—— mientras caminaba
mee-ehn-trahs kah-mee-**nah**-bah

—— while running

—— mientras corria
mee-ehn-trahs koh-**rhee**-ah

—— while playing sports

—— mientras jugaba deportes
mee-ehn-trahs hoo-**gah**-bah deh-**pohr**-tehs

—— while skating

—— mientras patinaba
mee-ehn-trahs pah-tee-**nah**-bah

Did he / she twist the elbow?

¿Se torció el codo?
Seh tohr-**see-oh** ehl **koh**-doh?

Did he / she drop something on his / her elbow?

¿Se le cayó algo encima del codo?
Seh leh kah-**yoh** ahl-goh ehn-**see**-mah dehl **koh**-doh?

What was it?

¿Qué fué?
Keh fweh?

___ A weight

___ Una pesa
Oo-nah **peh**-sah

___ A drawer

___ Un cajón
Oon kah-**hohn**

___ A book

___ Un libro
Oon lee-broh

Did he receive a blow to the elbow?

¿Recibió un golpe al codo?
Reh-see-**bee-oh** oon **gohl-peh** ahl **koh**-doh?

What was it?

¿Qué fué?
Keh fweh?

___ A baseball bat

___ Un bate de béisbol
Oon bah-teh deh **beh**-ees-bohl

___ A baseball

___ Una bola de béisbol
Oo-nah boh-lah deh **beh**-ees-bohl

___ A kick

___ Una patada
Oo-nah pah-**tah**-dah

Does he / she have swelling?

¿Tiene hinchazón?
Tee-eh-neh een-chah-**sohn?**

Does he / she have numbness in the elbow / arm?

¿Tiene entumido el codo / brazo?
Tee-eh-neh ehn-too-**mee**-doh ehl **koh**-doh / **brah**-soh?

Does he / she have weakness in the elbow / arm?

¿Tiene debilidad en el codo / brazo?

Tee-eh-neh deh-bee-lee-**dahd** ehn ehl **koh**-doh / **brah**-soh?

Does he / she have redness in the elbow / arm?

¿Tiene el codo / brazo rojo?

Tee-eh-neh ehl **koh**-doh / **brah**-soh **roh**-ho?

Does he / she have fever?

¿Tiene fiebre?

Tee-eh-neh **fee-eh**-breh?

Did he / she take medicine for the pain?

¿Tomó medicina para el dolor?

Toh-**moh** meh-dee-**see**-nah pah-rah ehl doh-**lohr?**

When?

¿Cuándo?

Kwahn-doh?

Common Terms for Elbow Pain

I am going to examine his / her elbow.

Voy a examinar su codo.

Boy ah eg-sah-mee-**nahr** soo **koh**-doh.

Extend the elbow.

Extiende el codo.

Egs-tee-**ehn**-deh ehl **koh**-doh.

Bend the elbow.

Doble el codo.

Doh-bleh ehl **koh**-doh.

Tell me if it hurts when I touch you here.

Dígame si le duele cuando le toco aquí.

Dee-gah-meh see leh dweh-leh **kwahn**-doh leh toh-koh ah-**kee**.

He / she needs an X-ray.

Necesita una radiografía.

Neh-seh-**see**-tah **oo**-nah **rah**-dee-oh-grah-**fee-ah.**

He / she has a fracture.

Tiene una fractura.
Tee-eh-neh **oo**-nah frag-**too**-rah.

He / she has a sprain.

Tiene una torcedura.
Tee-eh-neh **oo**-nah tohr-seh-**doo**-rah.

He / she has a skin infection.

Tiene una infección de la piel.
Tee-eh-neh **oo**-nah een-feg-**see-ohn** deh lah pee-ehl.

He / she has a contusion.

Tiene una contusión.
Tee-eh-neh **oo**-nah kohn-too-**see-ohn**.

He / she has a dislocation.

Tiene una luxación.
Tee-eh-neh **oo**-nah looks-ah-**see-ohn**.

He / she needs a cast
(posterior mold).

Necesita yeso.
Neh-seh-**see**-tah **yeh**-soh.

He / she needs antibiotics.

Necesita antibióticos.
Neh-seh-**see**-tah ahn-tee-bee-**oh**-tee-kohs.

He / she needs to see a bone specialist.

Él / ella necesita ver al especialista de los huesos.
Ehl / eh-yah neh-seh-**see**-tah behr ahl ehs-**peh-see**-ah-lees-tah deh los **weh**-sohs.

He / she needs surgery
(operation).

Él / ella necesita cirugía (operación).
Ehl / eh-yah neh-seh-**see**-tah see-roo-**hee**-ah (oh-peh-rah-**see-ohn**).

Discharge Instructions for Elbow Pain

Do not remove the posterior mold.

No se quite el yeso.
Noh seh kee-teh ehl **yeh**-soh.

Elevate his / her arm as much as possible.

Eleve su brazo lo más que sea posible.
Eh-**leh**-beh soo **brah**-soh loh mahs **keh** seh-ah poh-**see**-bleh.

Put ice on his / her elbow for twenty minutes every six hours for two days.

Ponga hielo en su codo por veinte minutos cada seis horas por dos días.
Pohn-gah **yeh**-loh ehn soo **koh**-doh pohr beh-**een**-teh mee-**noo**-tohs kah-dah says **oh**-rahs pohr dohs **dee**-ahs.

See the specialist on ___ at ___ o'clock.

Vaya con el especialista el día ___ a la hora ___ .
Bah-yah kohn ehl ehs-**peh-see**-ah-lees-tah ehl **dee**-ah ___ ah lah **oh**-rah ___ .

Give him / her Tylenol or Advil for pain every ___ hours.

Déle Tylenol o Advil para el dolor cada ___ horas.
Deh-leh Tay-leh-nohl oh Ad-beel pah-rah ehl doh-**lohr** kah-dah ___ **oh**-rahs.

Shoulder Pain / Trauma

Dolor de Hombro / Trauma

Doh-**lohr** deh **ohm**-broh / trah-oo-mah

When did the pain start?

¿Cuándo empezó el dolor?
Kwahn-doh ehm-peh-**soh** ehl doh-**lohr?**

___ Today

___ Hoy
Oy

___ Yesterday

___ Ayer
Ah-**yehr**

___ Days ago

Hace ___ días
Ah-seh **dee**-ahs

Did he / she fall . . . ?

¿Se cayó . . . ?
Seh kah-**yoh** . . . ?

___ while walking

___ mientras caminaba
mee-ehn-trahs kah-mee-**nah**-bah

___ while running

___ mientras corria
mee-ehn-trahs koh-**rhee**-ah

___ while playing sports

___ mientras jugaba deportes
mee-ehn-trahs hoo-**gah**-bah deh-**pohr**-tehs

___ while skating

___ mientras patinaba
mee-ehn-trahs pah-tee-**nah**-bah

Did he / she twist the shoulder?

¿Se torció el hombro?
Seh tohr-**see-oh** ehl **ohm**-broh?

Did he / she drop something on his / her shoulder?

¿Se le cayó algo encima del hombro?
Seh leh kah-**yoh** ahl-goh ehn-**see**-mah dehl **ohm**-broh?

What was it?

¿Qué fué?
Keh fweh?

— A weight

— Una pesa
Oo-nah **peh**-sah

— A drawer

— Un cajón
Oon kah-**hohn**

— A book

— Un libro
Oon lee-broh

Did he / she receive a blow to the shoulder?

¿Recibió un golpe al hombro?
Reh-see-**bee-oh** oon **gohl**-peh ahl **ohm**-broh?

What was it?

¿Qué fué?
Keh fweh?

— A baseball bat

— Un bate de béisbol
Oon bah-teh deh **beh**-ees-bohl

— A baseball

— Una bola de béisbol
Oo-nah boh-lah deh **beh**-ees-bohl

— A kick

— Una patada
Oo-nah pah-**tah**-dah

Does he / she have swelling?

¿Tiene hinchazón?
Tee-eh-neh een-chah-**sohn?**

Does he / she have numbness in the shoulder / arm?

¿Tiene entumido el hombro / brazo?
Tee-eh-neh ehn-too-**mee**-doh ehl **ohm**-broh / **brah**-soh?

Does he / she have weakness in the shoulder / arm?

¿Tiene debilidad en el hombro / brazo?
Tee-eh-neh deh-bee-lee-**dahd** ehn ehl **ohm**-broh / **brah**-soh?

Does he / she have redness in the shoulder?	¿Tiene el hombro rojo? **Tee-eh**-neh ehl **ohm**-broh **roh**-ho?
Does he / she have fever?	¿Tiene fiebre? **Tee-eh**-neh **fee-eh**-breh?
Did he / she take medicine for the pain?	¿Tomó medicina para el dolor? Toh-**moh** meh-dee-**see**-nah pah-rah ehl doh-**lohr?**
When?	¿Cuándo? **Kwahn**-doh?

Common Terms for Shoulder Pain

I am going to examine his / her shoulder.	Voy a examinar su hombro. Boy ah eg-sah-mee-**nahr** soo **ohm**-broh.
Tell me if it hurts when I touch you here.	Dígame si le duele cuando le toco aquí. **Dee**-gah-meh see leh dweh-leh **kwahn**-doh leh toh-koh ah-**kee.**
He / she needs an X-ray.	Necesita una radiografía. Neh-seh-**see**-tah **oo**-nah **rah**-dee-oh-grah-**fee-ah.**
He / she has a fracture.	Tiene una fractura. **Tee-eh**-neh **oo**-nah frag-**too**-rah.
He / she has a sprain.	Tiene una torcedura. **Tee-eh**-neh **oo**-nah tohr-seh-**doo**-rah.

He / she has a skin infection.

Tiene una infección de la piel.
Tee-eh-neh **oo**-nah een-feg-**see-ohn** deh lah pee-ehl.

He / she has a contusion.

Tiene una contusión.
Tee-eh-neh **oo**-nah kohn-too-**see-ohn**.

He / she has a dislocation.

Tiene una luxación.
Tee-eh-neh **oo**-nah looks-ah-**see-ohn**.

He / she needs an immobilizer.

Necesita un inmovilizador.
Neh-seh-**see**-tah oon een-moh-bee-lee-sah-**dohr.**

He / she needs antibiotics.

Necesita antibióticos.
Neh-seh-**see**-tah ahn-tee-bee-**oh**-tee-kohs.

He / she needs to see a bone specialist.

Él / ella necesita ver al especialista de los huesos.
Ehl / eh-yah neh-seh-**see**-tah behr ahl ehs-**peh-see**-ah-lees-tah deh los **weh**-sohs.

He / she needs surgery (operation).

Él / ella necesita cirugía (operación).
Ehl / eh-yah neh-seh-**see**-tah see-roo-**hee**-ah (oh-peh-rah-**see-ohn**).

Discharge Instructions for Shoulder Pain

Do not remove the posterior mold.

No se quite el yeso.
Noh seh kee-teh ehl **yeh**-soh.

Rest his / her shoulder as much as possible.

Descanse su hombro lo más que sea posible.
Dehs-**kahn**-seh soo **ohm**-broh loh mahs **keh** seh-ah poh-**see**-bleh.

Put ice on his / her shoulder for twenty minutes every six hours for two days.

Ponga hielo en su hombro por veinte minutos cada seis horas por dos días.
Pohn-gah **yeh**-loh ehn soo **ohm**-broh pohr beh-**een**-teh mee-**noo**-tohs kah-dah says **oh**-rahs pohr dohs **dee**-ahs.

See the specialist on ___ at ___ o'clock.

Vaya con el especialista el día ___ a la hora ___ .
Bah-yah kohn ehl ehs-**pen**-**see**-ah-lees-tah ehl **dee**-ah ___ ah lah **oh**-rah ___ .

Give him / her Tylenol or Advil for pain every ___ hours.

Déle Tylenol o Advil para el dolor cada ___ horas.
Deh-leh Tay-leh-nohl oh Ad-beel pah-rah ehl doh-**lohr** kah-dah ___ **oh**-rahs.

Back Pain

Dolor de Espalda

Doh-**lohr** deh ehs-**pahl**-dah

When did the pain start?

¿Cuándo empezó el dolor?
Kwahn-doh ehm-peh-**soh** ehl doh-**lohr?**

___ Today

___ Hoy
Oy

___ Yesterday

___ Ayer
Ah-**yehr**

___ Days ago

Hace ___ días
Ah-seh **dee**-ahs

Did he / she fall . . . ?

¿Se cayó . . . ?
Seh kah-**yoh** . . . ?

___ while walking

___ mientras caminaba
mee-ehn-trahs kah-mee-**nah**-bah

___ while running

___ mientras corria
mee-ehn-trahs koh-**rhee**-ah

___ while playing sports

___ mientras jugaba deportes
mee-ehn-trahs hoo-**gah**-bah deh-**pohr**-tehs

___ while skating

___ mientras patinaba
mee-ehn-trahs pah-tee-**nah**-bah

___ from a bed

___ de una cama
deh **oo**-nah **kah**-mah

___ from a chair

___ de una silla
deh **oo**-nah **see**-yah

___ from the stairs

___ de las escaleras
deh lahs ehs-kah-**leh**-rahs

Did he / she receive a blow to the back?

¿Recibió un golpe a la espalda?
Reh-see-**bee-oh** oon **gohl**-peh a lah ehs-**pahl**-dah?

What was he / she hit with?

¿Con qué se pegó?
Kohn **keh** seh peh-**goh?**

___ A baseball bat

___ Un bate de béisbol
Oon bah-teh deh **beh**-ees-bohl

___ A baseball

___ Bola de béisbol
Boh-lah deh **beh**-ees-
bohl

___ A kick

___ Una patada
Oo-nah pah-**tah**-dah

___ A fist

___ Un puño
Oon **poo**-nyoh

___ A piece of metal

___ Una pieza de metal
Oo-nah pee-**eh**-sah deh
meh-**tahl**

Did he / she twist his / her
back?

¿Se torció la espalda?
Seh tohr-**see-oh** lah ehs-**pahl**-
dah?

Does the pain go down his /
her leg?

¿Le corre el dolor a la pierna?
Leh **koh**-rheh ehl doh-**lohr** ah
lah **pee-ehr**-nah?

Does he / she have weakness
in the leg?

¿Tiene debilidad en la pierna?
Tee-eh-neh deh-bee-lee-**dahd**
ehn lah **pee-ehr**-nah?

Does he / she have numbness
in the leg?

¿Tiene la pierna entumida?
Tee-eh-neh lah **pee-ehr**-nah
ehn-too-**mee**-dah?

Does he / she have problems
urinating?

¿Tiene problemas para orinar?
Tee-eh-neh proh-**bleh**-mahs
pah-rah oh-ree-**nahr?**

Does he / she have problems
defecating?

¿Tiene problemas al defecar?
Tee-eh-neh pro-**bleh**-mahs ahl
deh-feh-**kahr?**

Does he / she have blood in the urine?

¿Tiene sangre en la orina?
Tee-eh-neh **sahn**-greh ehn lah oh-**ree**-nah?

Does it burn when he / she urinates?

¿Le arde cuando orina?
Leh ahr-deh **kwahn**-doh oh-**ree**-nah?

Is he / she urinating more than normal?

¿Está orinando más de lo normal?
Ehs-**tah** oh-ree-**nahn**-doh mahs deh loh nohr-**mahl?**

Does he / she have fever?

¿Tiene fiebre?
Tee-eh-neh **fee-eh**-breh?

Does he / she have trouble walking?

¿Tiene problemas para caminar?
Tee-eh-neh proh-**bleh**-mahs pah-rah kah-mee-**nahr?**

Does he / she have vomiting?

¿Tiene vómito?
Tee-eh-neh **boh**-mee-toh?

Does he / she have a cough?

¿Tiene tos?
Tee-eh-neh tohs?

Does he / she have shortness of breath?

¿Tiene falta de aire?
Tee-eh-neh fahl-tah deh ay-reh?

Common Terms During the Exam for Back Pain

Point to where you have the pain.

Apunte a dónde tiene el dolor.
Ah-**poon**-teh ah **dohn**-deh **tee-eh**-neh ehl doh-**lohr.**

Raise your left leg.

Levante la pierna izquierda.
Leh-**bahn**-teh lah **pee-ehr**-nah ees-**kee-ehr**-dah.

Raise your right leg.

Levante la pierna derecha.
Leh-**bahn**-teh lah **pee-ehr**-nah
deh-**reh**-chah.

Stand up straight.

Párese derecho.
Pah-reh-seh deh-**reh**-choh.

Bend over and touch your
toes.

Dóblese y toque los dedos de
los pies.
Doh-bleh-seh ee toh-keh lohs
deh-dohs deh lohs pee-ehs.

Lean backwards.

Inclínese hacia atrás.
Een-**klee**-neh-seh **ah**-see-ah
ah-**trahs.**

Do not bend your knees.

No doble las rodillas.
Noh doh-bleh lahs roh-**dee**-
yahs.

Bend to your right side.

Dóblese al lado derecho.
Doh-bleh-seh ahl lah-doh deh-
reh-choh.

Bend to your left side.

Dóblese al lado izquierdo.
Doh-bleh-seh ahl lah-doh ees-
kee-ehr-doh.

Turn your back to the right.

Voltea tu espalda al lado
derecho.
Bohl-**teh**-ah too ehs-**pahl**-dah
ahl lah-doh deh-**reh**-choh.

Turn your back to the left.

Voltea tu espalda al lado
izquierdo.
Bohl-**teh**-ah too ehs-**pahl**-dah
ahl lah-doh ees-**kee-ehr**-doh.

Tell me if you have pain when
I touch you.

Dígame si tiene dolor cuando
la / lo toco.
Dee-gah-meh see **tee-eh**-neh
doh-**lohr kwahn**-doh lah / loh
toh-koh.

Walk straight.	Camine derecho. Kah-**mee**-neh deh-**reh**-choh.
He / she needs an X-ray.	Él / ella necesita una radiografía. Ehl / eh-yah neh-seh-**see**-tah **oo**-nah **rah**-dee-oh-grah-**fee-ah.**
He / she needs a urine test.	Él / ella necesita una prueba de orina. Ehl / eh-yah neh-seh-**see**-tah **oo**-nah **proo-eh**-bah deh oh-**ree**-nah.
He / she has muscular pain.	Él / ella tiene dolor muscular. Ehl / eh-yah **tee-eh**-neh doh-**lohr** moos-koo-**lahr.**
He / she has a urinary tract infection.	Él / ella tiene una infección de la orina. Ehl / eh-yah **tee-eh**-neh **oo**-nah een-feg-**see-ohn** deh lah oh-**ree**-nah.
He / she has a fracture of a vertebra.	Él / ella tiene una fractura de su vértebra. Ehl / eh-yah **tee-eh**-neh **oo**-nah frag-**too**-rah deh soo **behr**-teh-brah.
He / she has back spasm.	Él / ella tiene espasmo de la espalda. Ehl / eh-yah **tee-eh**-neh ehs-**pahs**-moh deh lah ehs-**pahl**-dah.

Discharge Instructions for Back Pain

He / she needs to rest for a day.	Él / ella necesita estar de reposo por un día. Ehl / eh-yah neh-seh-**see**-tah ehs-**tahr** deh reh-**poh**-soh pohr oon **dee**-ah.

Put ice on his / her back for
half an hour every six hours
for two days.

Póngase hielo en la espalda
por media hora cada seis horas
por dos días.
Pohn-gah-seh **yeh**-loh ehn lah
ehs-**pahl**-dah pohr **meh**-dee-
ah **oh**-rah kah-dah says **oh**-
rahs pohr dohs **dee**-ahs.

Give him / her Tylenol or
Advil for pain every ___
hours

Déle Tylenol o Advil para el
dolor cada ___ horas.
Deh-leh Tay-leh-nohl oh Ad-
beel pah-rah ehl doh-**lohr** kah-
dah ___ **oh**-rahs.

Return to the hospital if he /
she has . . .

Regrese al hospital si él / ella
tiene . . .
Reh-**greh**-seh ahl **ohs**-pee-tahl
see ehl / eh-yah **tee-eh**-
neh . . .

___ worsening back pain

___ peor dolor de espalda
peh-**ohr** doh-**lohr** deh
ehs-**pahl**-dah

___ weakness in the leg

___ debilidad en la pierna
deh-bee-lee-**dahd** ehn
lah **pee-ehr**-nah

___ numbness in the leg

___ la pierna entumida
lah **pee-ehr**-nah ehn-too-
mee-dah

___ problems urinating or
defecating

___ problemas al orinar u
obrar
proh-**bleh**-mahs ahl oh-
ree-**nahr** u oh-**brahr**

Obstetrics/Gynecology

Vaginal Discharge

Deshecho Vaginal

Dehs-**eh**-choh bah-hee-**nahl**

How long has she had the discharge?

¿Cuánto tiempo tiene con el deshecho (flujo)?

Kwahn-toh **tee-ehm**-poh **tee-eh**-neh kohn ehl dehs-**eh**-choh (**floo**-hoh)?

What color is the discharge?

¿De qué color es el deshecho?

Deh **keh** koh-**lohr** ehs ehl dehs-**eh**-choh?

___ White

___ Blanco

Blahn-koh

___ Yellow

___ Amarillo

Ah-mah-**ree**-yoh

___ Brown

___ Café

Kah-**feh**

Does she have itching?

¿Tiene comezón?

Tee-eh-neh koh-meh-**sohn?**

Does the discharge have a bad odor?

¿Tiene mal olor el deshecho?

Tee-eh-neh mahl oh-**lohr** ehl dehs-**eh**-choh?

Does she have abdominal pain?

¿Tiene dolor abdominal?

Tee-eh-neh doh-**lohr** ab-doh-mee-**nahl?**

Does she have fever?

¿Tiene fiebre?

Tee-eh-neh **fee-eh**-breh?

Does she have burning when she urinates?

¿Tiene ardor al orinar?

Tee-eh-neh ahr-**dohr** ahl oh-ree-**nahr?**

With how many people does she have sex?	¿Con cuántas personas tiene sexo? Kohn **kwahn**-tahs pehr-**soh**-nahs **tee-eh**-neh **seg**-soh?
Does she have a new boyfriend?	¿Tiene un novio nuevo? **Tee-eh**-neh oon **noh**-bee-oh **nweh**-boh?
Has she had vaginal infections?	¿Ha tenido infecciones vaginales? Ah teh-**nee**-doh een-feg-**see-oh**-nehs bah-hee-**nah**-lehs?
When was her last period?	¿Cuándo fué su última regla? **Kwahn**-doh **fweh** soo **ool**-tee-mah **reh**-glah?
How many times has she been pregnant?	¿Cuántas veces ha estado embarazada? **Kwahn**-tahs **beh**-sehs ah ehs-**tah**-doh ehm-bah-rah-**sah**-dah?
How many children does she have?	¿Cuántos niños tiene? **Kwahn**-tohs **nee**-nyohs **tee-eh**-neh?
Has she had venereal diseases in the past?	¿Ha tenido enfermedades venéreas en el pasado? Ah teh-**nee**-doh **ehn**-fehr-meh-**dah**-dehs beh-**neh**-reh-ahs ehn ehl pah-**sah**-doh?
___ Gonorrhea	___ Gonorrea Goh-noh-**rhe**-ah
___ Syphilis	___ Sífilis **See**-fee-lees
___ Trichomonas	___ Tricomonas Tree-koh-**moh**-nahs

___ Chlamydia

___ Clamidia
Klah-**mee**-dee-ah

___ Herpes

___ Herpes
Ehr-pehs

Does she use condoms?

¿Usa condones?
Oo-sah kohn-**doh**-nehs?

Is she allergic to penicillin, tetracycline, or sulfa?

¿Es alérgica a la penicilina, tetraciclina, o sulfa?
Ehs ah-**lehr**-hee-kah ah lah peh-nee-see-**lee**-nah, teh-trah-see-**klee**-nah, oh **sool**-fah?

Common Terms for Vaginal Discharge

I need to do a vaginal exam.

Necesito hacerle un examen vaginal.
Neh-seh-**see**-toh ah-**sehr**-leh oon eg-**sah**-mehn bah-hee-**nahl**.

I need to do vaginal cultures.

Necesito hacerle cultivos vaginales.
Neh-seh-**see**-toh ah-**sehr**-leh kool-**tee**-bohs bah-hee-**nah**-lehs.

She has . . .

Ella tiene . . .
Eh-yah **tee-eh**-neh . . .

___ yeast (candida)

___ hongos (candida)
ohn-gohs (kahn-**dee**-dah)

___ chlamydia

___ clamidia
klah-**mee**-dee-ah

___ gardnerella

___ gardnerella
    gahrd-neh-**reh**-lah

___ trichomonas

___ tricomonas
    tree-koh-**moh**-nahs

___ pelvic inflammatory
    disease

___ enfermedad inflamatoria
    de la pelvis
    ehn-fehr-meh-**dahd** een-
    flah mah **toh** roo-ah deh
    lah **pehl**-bees

She is going to receive an
injection.

Ella va a recibir una inyección.
Eh-yah bah ah reh-see-**beer**
oo-nah een-jeg-**see-ohn.**

She needs intravenous
antibiotics.

Ella necesita antibióticos
intravenosos.
Eh-yah neh-seh-**see**-tah ahn-
tee-bee-**oh**-tee-kohs een-trah-
beh-**noh**-sohs.

We are going to admit her.

Vamos a internarla.
Bah-mohs ah **een**-tehr-**nahr**-
lah.

Discharge Instructions for Vaginal Discharge

Use the cream every night
before going to bed.

Use la crema todas las noches
antes de acostarse.
Oo-seh lah **kreh**-mah toh-dahs
lahs **noh**-chehs **ahn**-tehs deh
ah-kohs-**tahr**-seh.

Take a pill every ___ hours.

Tome una pastilla cada
___ horas.
Toh-meh **oo**-nah pahs-**tee**-yah
kah-dah ___ **oh**-rahs.

Use condoms.

Use condones.
Oo-seh kohn-**doh**-nehs.

Don't have sex for two weeks.

No tenga sexo por dos semanas.
Noh **tehn**-gah **seg**-soh pohr dohs seh-**mah**-nahs.

She must inform her boyfriends of her condition.

Debe de informarles a sus novios de su condición.
Deh-beh deh een-fohr-**mahr**-lehs ah soos **noh**-bee-ohs deh soo kohn-dee-**see-ohn**.

Her partner must also receive medical treatment.

Su pareja también debe de recibir tratamiento médico.
Soo pah-**reh**-hah tahm-bee-**ehn** deh-beh deh reh-see-**beer** trah-tah-mee-**ehn**-toh **meh**-dee-koh.

Vaginal Bleeding

Sangrado Vaginal

Sahn-**grah**-doh bah-hee-**nahl**

When was her last period or menstruation?

¿Cuándo fué su última regla o menstruación?
Kwahn-doh **fweh** soo **ool**-tee-mah **reh**-glah oh mehns-troo-ah-**see-ohn?**

___ Month ___ Day

___ Year

___ Mes   ___ Día
Mehs   **Dee**-ah

___ Año
Ah-nyoh

Is she pregnant?

¿Está embarazada?
Ehs-**tah** ehm-bah-rah-**sah**-dah?

How many months?

¿Cuántos meses?
Kwahn-tohs **meh**-sehs?

How many times has she been pregnant?

¿Cuántas veces ha estado embarazada?
Kwahn-tahs **beh**-sehs ah ehs-**tah**-doh ehm-bah-rah-**sah**-dah?

How many times has she delivered?

¿Cuántas veces ha dado a luz?
Kwahn-tahs **beh**-sehs ah dah-doh ah loos?

How many premature babies did she have?

¿Cuántos bebés prematuros tuvo?
Kwahn-tohs beh-**behs** preh-mah-**too**-rohs **too**-boh?

How many spontaneous abortions has she had?

¿Cuántos abortos espontáneos ha tenido?
Kwahn-tohs ah-**bohr**-tohs ehs-pohn-**tah**-neh-ohs ah teh-**nee**-doh?

How many induced abortions has she had?

¿Cuántos abortos provocados ha tenido?
Kwahn-tohs ah-**bohr**-tohs proh-boh-**kah**-dohs ah teh-**nee**-doh?

How many living children does she have?

¿Cuántos niños vivos tiene?
Kwahn-tohs **nee**-nyohs **bee**-bohs **tee-eh**-neh?

For how long has she had vaginal bleeding?

¿Por cuánto tiempo ha tenido sangrado vaginal?
Pohr **kwahn**-toh **tee-ehm**-poh ah teh-**nee**-doh sahn-**grah**-doh bah-hee-**nahl?**

Did it happen after a fall?

¿Ocurrió después de caerse?
Oh-koo-**rhee-oh** des-**pwehs**
deh kah-**ehr**-seh?

Did it happen after having
sex?

¿Ocurrió después de tener
relaciones sexuales?
Oh-koo-**rhee-oh** dehs-**pwehs**
deh teh-**nehr** reh-lah-**see-oh**-
nehs seg-soo-**ah**-lehs?

Did it happen after douching?

¿Ocurrió después de usar una
ducha vaginal?
Oh-koo-**rhee-oh** dehs-**pwehs**
deh **oo**-sahr **oo**-nah **doo**-chah
bah-hee-**nahl?**

Is the vaginal bleeding
constant?

¿Es el sangrado vaginal
constante?
Ehs ehl sahn-**grah**-doh bah-
hee-**nahl** kohns-**tahn**-teh?

Does the vaginal bleeding
come and go?

¿Le va y viene el sangrado
vaginal?
Leh bah ee bee-eh-neh ehl
sahn-**grah**-doh bah-hee-**nahl?**

Has she passed blood clots?

¿Ha arrrojado coágulos de
sangre?
Ah ah-rho-**ha**-doh koh-**ah**-goo-
lohs deh **sahn**-greh?

Has she passed tissue?

¿Ha pasado carnosidad o
tejido?
Ah pah-**sah**-doh kahr-noh-see-
dad oh teh-**hee**-doh?

How many sanitary pads did
she use today?

¿Cuántas toallas femininas usó
hoy?
Kwahn-tahs toh-**ah**-yahs feh-
mee-**nee**-nahs oo-**soh** oy?

Does she have pain in the belly or stomach?	¿Tiene dolor en el vientre o estómago? **Tee-eh**-neh doh-**lohr** ehn ehl bee-**ehn**-treh oh ehs-**toh**-mah-goh?
Is the pain constant?	¿Es el dolor constante? Ehs ehl doh-**lohr** kohns-**tahn**-teh?
Does the pain come and go?	¿Le va y viene el dolor? Leh bah ee bee-eh-neh ehl doh-**lohr?**
How long does the pain last for?	¿Cuánto tiempo le dura el dolor? **Kwahn**-toh **tee-ehm**-poh leh **doo**-rah ehl doh-**lohr?**
Does the pain stay in one place?	¿Se queda el dolor en un solo lugar? Seh **keh**-dah ehl doh-**lohr** ehn oon soh-loh loo-**gahr?**
Does the pain travel to another place?	¿Le viaja el dolor a otro lado? Leh bee-**ah**-ha ehl doh-**lohr** ah oh-troh lah-doh?
Does she have cramps in the belly?	¿Tiene calambres o retortijones en el vientre? **Tee-eh**-neh kah-**lahm**-brehs oh reh-tohr-tee-**ho**-nehs ehn ehl bee-**ehn**-treh?
Does she have nausea or vomiting?	¿Tiene náusea o vómito? **Tee-eh**-neh nah-**oo**-seh-ah oh **boh**-mee-toh?
Does she have diarrhea?	¿Tiene diarrea? **Tee-eh**-neh dee-ah-**rhe-ah?**

Does she have a fever?	¿Tiene fiebre? **Tee-eh**-neh **fee-eh**-breh?
Does she feel dizzy?	¿Se siente mareada? Seh **see-ehn**-teh mah-reh-**ah**-dah?
Does she have back pain?	¿Tiene dolor en la espalda? **Tee-eh**-neh doh-**lohr** ehn-lah ehs-**pahl**-dah?
Does she have a vaginal discharge?	¿Tiene flujo vaginal? **Tee-eh**-neh **floo**-ho bah-hee-**nahl?**
What color is it?	¿De qué color es? Deh **keh** koh-**lohr** ehs?
___ Yellow	___ Amarilla Ah-mah-**ree**-yah
___ White	___ Blanca **Blahn**-kah
___ Brown	___ Café Kah-**feh**
Is she urinating more than normal?	¿Está orinando más de lo normal? Ehs-**tah** oh-ree-**nahn**-doh mahs deh loh nohr-**mahl?**
Does she have burning when she urinates?	¿Tiene ardor al orinar? **Tee-eh**-neh ahr-**dohr** ahl oh-ree-**nahr?**
Does she have pain when she urinates?	¿Tiene dolor al orinar? **Tee-eh**-neh doh-**lohr** ahl oh-ree-**nahr?**

Is she allergic to any medicine or food?

¿Es alérgica a alguna medicina o alimento?
Ehs ah-**lehr**-hee-kah ah ahl-**goo**-nah meh-dee-**see**-nah oh ah-lee-**mehn**-toh?

What medicine has she taken for the pain?

¿Qué medicina ha tomado para el dolor?
Keh meh-dee-**see**-nah ah toh-**mah**-doh pah-rah ehl doh-**lohr?**

Does she have or suffer from . . . ?

Ella tiene o ha padecido de . . . ?
Eh-yah **tee-eh**-neh oh ah pah-deh-**see**-doh deh . . . ?

___ anemia

___ anemia
ah-**neh**-mee-ah

___ diabetes

___ diabetes
dee-ah-**beh**-tehs

___ heart disease

___ enfermedad del corazón
ehn-fehr-meh-**dad** dehl koh-rah-**sohn**

___ kidney disease

___ enfermedad del riñón
ehn-fehr-meh-**dad** dehl ree-**nyohn**

At what age did she start having her periods?

¿A los cuántos años comenzó a reglar o menstruar?
Ah lohs **kwahn**-tohs **ah**-nyohs koh-mehn-**soh** ah reh-**glahr** oh mehns-troo-**ahr?**

Are her periods regular?

¿Son regulares sus reglas o menstruaciones?
Sohn reh-goo-**lah**-rehs soos **reh**-glahs oh mehns-troo-ah-**see-oh**-nehs?

Has she ever had . . . ?

Alguna vez ha tenido . . . ?
Ahl-**goo**-nah behs ah teh-**nee**-doh . . . ?

—— gonorrhea

—— gonorrea
goh-noh-**rhe**-ah

—— infection in a tube

—— infección en un tubo
een-feg-**see-ohn** ehn oon **too**-boh

—— syphilis

—— sífilis
see-fee-lees

—— pelvic infection

—— infección pélvica
een-feg-**see-ohn pehl**-bee-kah

—— herpes

—— herpes
ehr-pehs

—— chlamydia

—— clamidia
klah-**mee**-dee-ah

What kind of contraceptive does she use to prevent pregnancy?

¿Qué clase de anticonceptivo usa para prevenir el embarazo?
Keh klah-seh deh **ahn**-tee-kohn-sep-**tee**-boh **oo**-sah pah-rah preh-beh-**neer** ehl ehm-bah-**rah**-soh?

—— Nothing

—— Nada
Nah-dah

—— Condoms

—— Condones
Kohn-**doh**-nehs

—— Pills

—— Pastillas
Pahs-**tee**-yhahs

—— Intrauterine device

—— Dispositivo intrauterino
Dees-poh-see-**tee**-boh een-trah-oo-teh-**ree**-noh

Has she ever had a pregnancy in the tube?

¿Alguna vez ha tenido un embarazo en un tubo?
Ahl-**goo**-nah behs ah teh-**nee**-doh oon ehm-bah-**rah**-soh ehn oon **too**-boh?

Common Terms During the Exam for Vaginal Bleeding

I am going to examine your abdomen.

Voy a examinar su abdomen.
Boy ah eg-sah-mee-**nahr** soo ab-**doh**-mehn.

I need to do a rectal exam.

Necesito hacerle un examen del recto.
Neh-seh-**see**-toh ah-**sehr**-leh oon eg-**sah**-mehn dehl **reg**-toh.

I need to do a genital exam.

Necesito hacerle un examen genital.
Neh-seh-**see**-toh ah-**sehr**-leh oon eg-**sah**-mehn he-nee-**tahl.**

I need to do a pelvic exam.

Necesito hacerle un examen pélvico.
Neh-seh-**see**-toh ah-**sehr**-leh oon eg-**sah**-mehn **pehl**-bee-koh.

Bend your knees.

Doble las rodillas.
Doh-bleh lahs roh-**dee**-yhahs.

Separate your knees.

Separe las rodillas.
Seh-**pah**-reh lahs roh-**dee**-yhahs.

Do you have pain when I touch here?

¿Tiene dolor cuando le toco aquí?
Tee-eh-neh doh-**lohr kwahn**-doh leh toh-koh ah-**kee?**

We need to do blood and urine tests.

Necesitamos hacerle pruebas de sangre y orina.
Neh-seh-see-**tah**-mohs ah-**sehr**-leh **proo-eh**-bahs deh **sahn**-greh ee oh-**ree**-nah.

She needs an ultrasound.

Ella necesita un ultrasonido.
Eh-yah neh-seh-**see**-tah oon **ool**-trah-soh-**nee**-doh.

She needs an operation.

Ella necesita una operación.
Eh-yah neh-seh-**see**-tah **oo**-nah oh-peh-rah-**see-ohn.**

She is (is not) pregnant.

Ella está (no está) embarazada.
Eh-yah ehs-**tah** (noh ehs-**tah**) ehm-bah-rah-**sah**-dah.

She has an ectopic pregnancy.

Ella tiene el embarazo en un tubo.
Eh-yah **tee-eh**-neh ehl ehm-bah-**rah**-soh ehn oon **too**-boh.

She has a threatened abortion.

Ella tiene una amenaza de aborto.
Eh-yah **tee-eh**-neh **oo**-nah ah-meh-**nah**-sah deh ah-**bohr**-toh.

She has a normal pregnancy.

Ella tiene un embarazo normal.
Eh-yah **tee-eh**-neh oon ehm-bah-**rah**-soh nohr-**mahl.**

Discharge Instructions for Vaginal Bleeding

Return in two days to repeat her blood test.

Regrese en dos días para repetir su examen de sangre.
Reh-**greh**-seh ehn dohs **dee**-ahs pah-rah reh-peh-**teer** soo eg-**sah**-mehn deh **sahn**-greh.

Avoid sex, vaginal douching, or tampons.

Evite el sexo, duchas vaginales, o tampones.

Eh-**bee**-teh ehl **seg**-soh, **doo**-chahs bah-hee-**nah**-lehs oh tahm-**poh**-nehs.

Return at once if she passes tissue or if bleeding worsens.

Regrese pronto si ella pasa tejido (carnosidad) o si el sangrado aumenta.

Reh-**greh**-seh **prohn**-toh see eh-yah pah-sah teh-**hee**-doh (kahr-noh-see-**dahd**) oh see ehl sahn-**grah**-doh ah-oo-**mehn**-tah.

Return if she has fever or abdominal pain.

Regrese si tiene fiebre o dolor abdominal.

Reh-**greh**-seh see **tee-eh**-neh **fee-eh**-breh oh doh-**lohr** ab-doh-mee-**nahl**.

Return if she has dizziness or headache.

Regrese si tiene mareos o dolor de cabeza.

Reh-**greh**-seh see **tee-eh**-neh mah-**reh**-ohs oh doh-**lohr** deh kah-**beh**-sah.

Labor Pains

Dolores de Parto

Doh-**loh**-rehs deh **pahr**-toh

When did the pain start?

¿Cuándo empezó el dolor?
Kwahn-doh ehm-peh-**soh** ehl doh-**lohr?**

It has been ___ hours	Hace ___ horas
	Ah-seh **oh**-rahs
___ days	___ días
	dee-ahs

Do you have pain in the back?	¿Tiene dolor en la espalda?
	Tee-eh-neh doh-**lohr** ehn lah ehs-**pahl**-dah?

Do you have pain in the abdomen?	¿Tiene dolor en el abdomen?
	Tee-eh-neh doh-**lohr** ehn ehl ab-**doh**-mehn?

Do you have contractions?	¿Tiene contracciones?
	Tee-eh-neh kohn-trahk-**see-ohn**-ehs?

Every how many minutes do you have the contractions?	¿Cada cuántos minutos le vienen las contracciones?
	Kah-dah **kwahn**-tohs mee-**noo**-tohs leh bee-eh-nehn lahs kohn-trahk-**see-ohn**-ehs?

How many minutes do the contractions last?	¿Cuántos minutos le duran las contracciones?
	Kwahn-tohs mee-**noo**-tohs leh **doo**-rahn lahs kohn-trahk-**see-ohn**-ehs?

Do you having vaginal bleeding?	¿Tiene sangrado vaginal?
	Tee-eh-neh sahn-**grah**-doh bah-hee-**nahl?**

Did your bag of water break?	¿Se le rompió la fuente del agua?
	Seh leh rohm-pee-**oh** lah **fwehn**-teh dehl **ah**-gwah?

What color was the water?	¿De qué color fué el agua?
	Deh **keh** koh-**lohr fweh** ehl **ah**-gwah?

___ Clear

___ Clara
Klah-rah

___ Yellow

___ Amarilla
Ah-mah-ree-yah

___ Green

___ Verde
Behr-deh

___ Red

___ Roja
Roh-ha

When did your bag of water break?

¿Cuándo se le rompió la fuente del agua?
Kwahn-doh seh leh rohm-pee-oh lah fwehn-teh dehl ah-gwah?

When was your last period?

¿Cuándo fué su última regla?
Kwahn-doh fweh soo ool-tee-mah reh-glah?

___ Month ___ Day
___ Year

___ Mes ___ Día
Mehs Dee-ah
___ Año
Ah-nyoh

How many pregnancies have you had?

¿Cuántos embarazos ha tenido?
Kwahn-tohs ehm-bah-rah-sohs ah teh-nee-doh?

How many babies do you have?

¿Cuántos bebés tiene?
Kwahn-tohs beh-behs tee-eh-neh?

Have you received prenatal care?

¿Ha recibido cuidado prenatal?
Ah reh-see-bee-doh kwi-dah-doh preh-nah-tahl?

When was the last time you visited the doctor?

¿Cuándo fué la última vez que visitó a su médico?
Kwahn-doh **fweh** lah **ool**-tee-mah behs **keh** bee-see-**toh** ah soo **meh**-dee-koh?

Have you had infections during the pregnancy?

¿Ha tenido infecciones durante su embarazo?
Ah teh-**nee**-doh een-feg-**see-ohn**-ehs doo-**rahn**-teh soo ehm-bah-**rah**-soh?

___ Gonorrhea

___ Gonorrea
Goh-noh-**rhe**-ah

___ Urinary (bladder) infection

___ Infección urinaria (de la vejiga)
Een-feg-**see-ohn** oo-ree-**nah**-ree-ah (deh lah beh-**hee**-gah)

___ Syphilis

___ Sífilis
See-fee-lees

___ Vaginal infection

___ Infección vaginal
Een-feg-**see-ohn** bah-hee-**nahl**

___ Herpes

___ Herpes
Ehr-pehs

___ Chlamydia

___ Clamidia
Klah-**mee**-dee-ah

Have you had problems with other pregnancies like . . . ?

¿Ha tenido problemas con los otros embarazos como . . . ?
Ah teh-**nee**-doh proh-**bleh**-mahs kohn lohs oh-trohs ehm-bah-**rah**-sohs **koh**-moh . . . ?

___ diabetes

___ diabetes
dee-ah-**beh**-tehs

___ high blood pressure

___ alta presión
ahl-tah preh-**see-ohn**

___ convulsions

___ convulsiones
kohn-bool-**see-oh**-nehs

___ premature births

___ partos prematuros
pahr-tohs preh-mah-**too**-rohs

Did you have your babies by vaginal delivery?

¿Tuvo sus bebés por parto vaginal?
Too-boh soos beh-**behs** pohr **pahr**-toh bah-hee-**nahl?**

Did you have your babies by C-section?

¿Tuvo sus bebés por cesárea?
Too-boh soos beh-**behs** pohr seh-**sah**-reh-ah?

Common Terms During the Exam for Labor Pains

I need to do a vaginal exam.

Necesito hacerle un examen vaginal.
Neh-seh-**see**-toh ah-**sehr**-leh oon eg-**sah**-mehn bah-hee-**nahl.**

Don't push.

No empuje.
Noh ehm-**poo**-heh.

Push.

Empuje.
Ehm-**poo**-heh

She is (you are) going to deliver.

Ella va (tú vas) a dar a luz (va a aliviarse).
Eh-yah bah (too bahs) ah dahr ah loos (bah ah ah-lee-**biarh**-seh).

I am going to put a monitor on her abdomen.

Voy a ponerle un monitor en su abdomen.
Boy ah poh-**nehr**-leh oon moh-nee-**tohr** ehn soo ab-**doh**-mehn.

I am going to listen to the baby's heartbeat.

Voy a escuchar los latidos del corazón del bebé.
Boy ah ehs-koo-**chahr** lohs lah-**tee**-dohs dehl koh-rah-**sohn** dehl beh-**beh.**

Her (your) cervix is not dilated yet.

Todavía su (tu) matriz no está dilatada.
Toh-dah-**bee**-ah soo (too) mah-**trees** noh ehs-**tah** dee-lah-**tah**-dah.

She is (you are) not in labor yet.

Todavía no va (vas) a tener el parto.
Toh-dah-**bee**-ah noh bah (bahs) ah teh-**nehr** ehl **pahr**-toh.

She needs (you need) an ultrasound to check the baby and the placenta.

Ella necesita (tú necesitas) un ultrasonido para revisar el bebé y la placenta.
Eh-yah neh-seh-**see**-tah (too neh-seh-**see**-tahs) oon **ool**-trah-soh-**nee**-doh pah-rah reh-bee-**sahr** ahl beh-**beh** ee lah plah-**sehn**-tah.

Discharge Instructions for Labor Pains

Return to the hospital if . . .

Regrese al hospital si . . .
Reh-**greh**-seh ahl **ohs**-pee-tahl see . . .

___ your bag of water breaks

___ se le rompe la fuente del agua
seh leh **rohm**-peh lah **fwehn**-teh dehl **ah**-gwah

___ your pains are more frequent and stronger

___ sus dolores son más seguidos y fuertes
soos doh-**loh**-rehs sohn mahs seh-**gee**-dohs ee **fwehr**-tehs

___ you have vaginal bleeding

___ tiene sangrado vaginal
tee-eh-neh sahn-**grah**-doh bah-hee-**nahl**

Rape / Sexual Assault

Violación / Asalto Sexual

Bee-oh-lah-**see-ohn** / Ah-**sahl**-toh seg-soo-**ahl**

Do you know who did it?

¿Sabe quien lo hizo?
Sah-beh kee-**ehn** loh **ee**-soh?

What time did it happen?

¿A qué hora ocurrió?
Ah **keh oh**-rah oh-koo-**rhee-oh?**

When did it happen?

¿Cuándo ocurrió?
Kwahn-doh oh-koo-**rhee-oh?**

How many men were there?

¿Cuántos hombres eran?
Kwahn-tohs **ohm**-brehs eh-rahn?

| Was there vaginal penetration? | ¿Hubo penetración de la vagina?
Oo-boh peh-neh-trah-**see-ohn** deh lah bah-**hee**-nah? |

| Was there rectal penetration? | ¿Hubo penetración del recto?
Oo-boh peh-neh-trah-**see-ohn** dehl **reg**-toh? |

| Was there oral penetration? | ¿Hubo penetración oral?
Oo-boh peh-neh-trah-**see-ohn** oh-**rahl?** |

| Does she know if the rapist used a condom? | ¿Sabe si el violador usó un condón?
Sah-beh see ehl bee-oh-lah-**dohr** oo-**soh** oon kohn-**dohn?** |

| Does she know if he ejaculated inside her? | ¿Sabe si él eyaculó dentro de ella?
Sah-beh see ehl eh-yhah-koo-**loh dehn**-troh deh eh-yah? |

| Did the rapist use any foreign objects? | ¿Usó el violador objetos extraños?
Oo-**soh** ehl bee-oh-lah-**dohr** ohb-**heh**-tohs egs-**trah**-nyohs? |

| Was she beaten? | ¿Fué golpeada?
Fweh gohl-peh-**ah**-dah? |

| Was she bitten? | ¿Fué mordida?
Fweh mohr-**dee**-dah? |

| Since the rape has she . . . ? | ¿Desde que fué violada se ha . . . ?
Dehs-deh **keh fweh** bee-oh-**lah**-dah seh ah . . . |

| ___ showered | ___ bañado
bah-**nyah**-doh |

___ changed clothes

___ cambiado la ropa
kahm-bee-**ah**-do lah **roh**-pah

___ brushed her teeth

___ lavado los dientes
lah-**bah**-doh lohs dee-**ehn**-tehs

___ urinated

___ orinado
oh-ree-**nah**-doh

___ defecated

___ obrado o defecado
oh-**brah**-doh oh deh-feh-**kah**-doh

When was her last period?

¿Cuándo fué su última regla?
Kwahn-doh **fweh** soo **ool**-tee-mah **reh**-glah?

Is she taking contraceptives?

¿Está tomando anticonceptivos?
Ehs-**tah** toh-**mahn**-doh ahn-tee-kohn-sehp-**tee**-bohs?

When was the last time she had sexual relations?

¿Cuándo fué la última vez que tuvo relaciones sexuales?
Kwahn-doh **fweh** lah **ool**-tee-mah behs **keh too**-boh reh-lah-**see-oh**-nehs seg-soo-**ah**-lehs?

Does she want me to call a friend or relative for her?

¿Quiere que le llame a una amistad o pariente?
Kee-**eh**-reh **keh** leh **yha**-meh ah **oo**-nah ah-mees-**tahd** oh pah-ree-**ehn**-teh?

Does she want to speak with the . . . ?

¿Quiere hablar con . . . ?
Kee-**eh**-reh ah-**blahr** kohn . . .

___ social worker

___ el (la) trabajador (ra) social
ehl (lah) trah-bah-ha-**dohr** (doh-rah) soh-see-ahl

___ psychiatrist

___ el psiquiatra
ehl see-kee-**ah**-trah

___ Rape Crisis Center

___ el centro de crisis para violaciones
ehl **sehn**-troh deh **kree**-sees pah-rah bee-oh-lah-**see-ohn**-ehs

Is she allergic to any antibiotic?

¿Es alérgica a algún antibiótico?
Ehs ah-**lehr**-hee-kah ah ahl-**goon** ahn-tee-bee-**oh**-tee-koh?

Common Terms During the Exam of the Rape Patient

We are going to do a blood and urine test.

Vamos a hacerle una prueba de orina y sangre.
Bah-mohs ah ah-**sehr**-leh **oo**-nah **proo-eh**-bah deh oh-**ree**-nah ee **sahn**-greh.

We need to collect some cultures.

Necesitamos hacer cultivos.
Neh-seh-see-**tah**-mohs ah-**sehr** kool-**tee**-bohs.

She will receive an injection and pills to prevent venereal diseases.

Recibirá una inyección y pastillas para prevenir enfermedades venéreas.
Reh-see-bee-**rah oo**-nah een-jeg-**see-ohn** ee pahs-**tee**-yhahs pah-rah preh-beh-**neer** ehn-fehr-meh-**dah**-dehs beh-**neh**-reh-ahs.

I need to give her pills to prevent the pregnancy.	Necesito darle pastillas para prevenir el embarazo. Neh-seh-**see**-toh dahr-leh pahs-**tee**-yhahs pah-rah preh-boh **neer** ohl ohm bah **rah** soh.

Discharge Instructions for Sexual Assault

Return to the hospital if she has . . .	Regrese al hospital si tiene . . . Reh-**greh**-seh ahl **ohs**-pee-tahl see **tee-eh**-neh . . .
___ vaginal bleeding	___ sangrado vaginal sahn-**grah**-doh bah-hee-**nahl**
___ vaginal discharge	___ deshecho o flujo vaginal dehs-**eh**-choh oh **floo**-ho bah-hee-**nahl**
___ burning on urination	___ ardor al orinar ahr-**dohr** ahl oh-ree-**nahr**
___ fever or vomiting	___ fiebre o vómito **fee-eh**-breh oh **boh**-mee-toh

Instructions for the Vitullo Kit

I need to comb her / your hair.	Necesito peinar su pelo. Neh-seh-**see**-toh peh-ee-**nahr** soo **peh**-loh.
I need to comb her / your pubic hair.	Necesito peinar su pelo púbico. Neh-seh-**see**-toh peh-ee-**nahr** soo **peh**-loh **poo**-bee-koh.

I need to do vaginal cultures.

Necesito hacer cultivos vaginales.
Neh-seh-**see**-toh ah-**sehr** kool-**tee**-vohs bah-hee-**nah**-lehs.

I need samples of her / your mouth and rectum.

Necesito muestras de su boca y recto.
Neh-seh-**see**-toh **mwehs**-trahs deh soo **boh**-kah ee **reg**-toh.

I need to clean under her / your fingernails.

Necesito limpiar debajo de sus uñas.
Neh-seh-**see**-toh leem-pee-**ahr** deh-**bah**-hoh deh soos **oo**-nyahs.

Can she / you leave her / your underwear for evidence?

¿Puede dejar su ropa interior como evidencia?
Pweh-deh deh-**har** soo **roh**-pah een-teh-ree-**ohr koh**-moh eh-bee-**dehn**-see-ah?

G

Genitourinary

Urinary Tract Infection

Infección Urinaria

Een-feg-**see-ohn** Oo-ree-**nah**-ree-ah

Is she urinating more than normal?

¿Está orinando más de lo normal?
Ehs-**tah** oh-ree-**nahn**-doh mahs deh loh nohr-**mahl?**

Does it burn when she urinates?

¿Le arde cuando orina?
Leh ahr-deh **kwahn**-doh oh-**ree**-nah?

Does she feel pressure over the bladder when she urinates?

¿Siente presión sobre la vejiga cuando orina?
See-ehn-teh preh-**see-ohn soh**-breh lah beh-**hee**-gah **kwahn**-doh oh-**ree**-nah?

Has she noticed blood in the urine?

¿Ha notado sangre en la orina?
Ah noh-**tah**-doh **sahn**-greh ehn lah oh-**ree**-nah?

Does she have nausea or vomiting?

¿Tiene náusea o vómito?
Tee-eh-neh **nah**-oo-seh-ah oh **boh**-mee-toh?

Does she have pain in the flank?

¿Tiene dolor en el costado?
Tee-eh-neh doh-**lohr** ehn ehl kohs-**tah**-doh?

Does she have abdominal pain?

¿Tiene dolor abdominal?
Tee-eh-neh doh-**lohr** ab-doh-mee-**nahl?**

Does she have a fever?

¿Tiene fiebre?
Tee-eh-neh **fee-eh**-breh?

Does her urine have a bad
odor?

¿Tiene mal olor su orina?
Tee-eh-neh mahl oh-**lohr** soo
oh-**ree**-nah?

Does she have a vaginal
discharge?

¿Tiene deshecho vaginal?
Tee-eh-neh dehs-**eh**-choh
bah-hee-**nahl?**

What color is the discharge?

¿De qué color es el deshecho?
Deh **keh** koh-**lohr** ehs ehl deh-
eh-choh?

___ Yellow

___ Amarillo
Ah-mah-**ree**-yoh

___ White

___ Blanco
Blahn-koh

___ Brown

___ Café
Kah-**feh**

Does she have vaginal itching?

¿Tiene comezón en la vagina?
Tee-eh-neh koh-meh-**sohn** ehn
lah bah-**hee**-nah?

When was her last normal
period?

¿Cuándo fué su última regla
normal?
Kwahn-doh **fweh** soo **ool**-tee-
mah **reh**-glah nohr-**mahl?**

Is she allergic to penicillin or
sulfa?

¿Es alérgica a la penicilina o
sulfa?
Ehs ah-**lehr**-hee-kah ah lah
peh-nee-see-**lee**-nah oh **sool**-
fah?

Does she suffer from . . . ?

¿Sufre ella de . . . ?
Soo-freh eh-yah deh . . . ?

—— chronic bladder
infections

—— infecciones crónicas de
la vejiga
een-feg-**see-oh**-nehs
kroh-nee-kahs deh lah
beh-**hee**-gah

—— kidney stones

—— cálculos de los riñones
kahl-koo-lohs deh lohs
ree-**nyoh**-nehs

—— diabetes

—— diabetes
dee-ah-**beh**-tehs

Common Terms for UTI

I need to do a urine test.

Necesito hacerle una prueba
de orina.
Neh-seh-**see**-toh ah-**sehr**-leh
oo-nah **proo-eh**-bah deh oh-
ree-nah.

She has a urinary tract
infection.

Ella tiene una infección de la
orina.
Eh-yah **tee-eh**-neh **oo**-nah
een-feg-**see-ohn** deh lah oh-
ree-nah.

She needs to take antibiotics
for the infection.

Necesita tomar antibióticos
para la infección.
Neh-seh-**see**-tah toh-**mahr**
ahn-tee-bee-**oh**-tee-kohs pah-
rah lah een-feg-**see-ohn**.

Discharge Instructions for UTI

Take the antibiotic every
___ hours.

Tome el antibiótico cada
___ horas.
Toh-meh ehl ahn-tee-bee-**oh**-tee-koh kah-dah ___ **oh**-rahs.

Drink plenty of liquids.

Tome muchos líquidos.
Toh-meh **moo**-chohs **lee**-kee-dohs.

Return to the hospital if she
has . . .

Regrese al hospital si
tiene . . .
Reh-**greh**-seh ahl **ohs**-pee-tahl see **tee-eh**-neh . . .

___ fever

___ fiebre
fee-eh-breh

___ vomiting

___ vómito
boh-mee-toh

___ abdominal pain

___ dolor abdominal
doh-**lohr** ab-doh-mee-**nahl**

Penile Discharge

Deshecho del Pene

Dehs-**eh**-choh dehl
peh-neh

For how many days have you
had the discharge?

¿Por cuántos días ha tenido el
deshecho?
Pohr **kwahn**-tohs **dee**-ahs ah
teh-**nee**-doh ehl dehs-**eh**-choh?

What color is the discharge?

¿De qué color es el deshecho?
Deh **keh** koh-**lohr** ehs ehl
dehs-**eh**-choh?

— Clear

— Claro
Klah-roh

— White

— Blanco
Blahn-koh

— Yellow

— Amarillo
Ah-mah-**ree**-yoh

Do you have burning when
you urinate?

¿Tiene ardor al orinar?
Tee-eh-neh ahr-**dohr** ahl oh-
ree-**nahr?**

Have you noticed blood in the
urine?

¿Ha notado sangre en su
orina?
Ah noh-**tah**-doh **sahn**-greh
ehn soo oh-**ree**-nah?

Do you have pain in the
testicles?

¿Tiene dolor en los testículos?
Tee-eh-neh doh-**lohr** ehn lohs
tehs-**tee-koo**-lohs?

Do you have abdominal pain?

¿Tiene dolor abdominal?
Tee-eh-neh doh-**lohr** abh-doh-
mee-**nahl?**

Do you have a fever?

¿Tiene fiebre?
Tee-eh-neh **fee-eh**-breh?

Have you had venereal
diseases in the past?

¿Ha tenido enfermedades
venéreas en el pasado?
Ah teh-**nee**-doh ehn-fehr-meh-
dah-dehs beh-**neh**-reh-ahs
ehn ehl pah-**sah**-doh?

— Gonorrhea

— Gonorrea
Goh-noh-**rhe**-ah

— Syphilis

— Sifilis
See-fee-lees

___ Trichomonas

___ Tricomonas
Tree-koh-**moh**-nahs

___ Chlamydia

___ Clamidia
Klah-**mee**-dee-ah

___ Herpes

___ Herpes
Ehr-pehs

With how many people do you have sex?

¿Con cuántas personas tiene sexo?
Kohn **kwahn**-tahs pehr-**soh**-nahs **tee-eh**-neh **seg**-soh?

Do you have a new girlfriend?

¿Tiene una novia nueva?
Tee-eh-neh **oo**-nah noh-**bee**-ah **nweh**-bah?

Do you have sexual relations with . . . ?

Tiene relaciones sexuales con . . . ?
Tee-eh-neh reh-lah-**see-oh**-nehs seg-soo-**ah**-lehs kohn . . . ?

___ men

___ hombres
ohm-brehs

___ women

___ mujeres
moo-**heh**-rehs

___ prostitutes

___ prostitutas
prohs-tee-**too**-tahs

Do you use condoms?

¿Usa condones?
Oo-sah kohn-**doh**-nehs?

Common Terms During the Exam for Penile Discharge

I need to examine your penis and testicles.	Necesito examinar su pene y testículos. Neh-seh-**see**-toh eg-sah-mee-**nahr** soo **peh**-neh ee tehs-**tee-koo**-lohs.
I need to do penile cultures.	Necesito hacerle cultivos del pene. Neh-seh-**see**-toh ah-**sehr**-leh kool-**tee**-bohs dehl **peh**-neh.
I need a urine sample.	Necesito una muestra de orina. Neh-seh-**see**-toh **oo**-nah **mwehs**-trah deh oh-**ree**-nah.
You have a venereal disease.	Tiene una enfermedad venérea. **Tee-eh**-neh **oo**-nah ehn-fehr-meh-**dahd** beh-**neh**-reh-ah.
I am going to give you an antibiotic injection.	Le voy a dar una inyección de antibiótico. Leh boy ah dahr **oo**-nah een-jeg-**see-ohn** deh ahn-tee-bee-**oh**-tee-koh.

Discharge Instructions for Penile Discharge

Inform all of your partners about your condition.	Informe a todas sus parejas acerca de su condición. Een-**fohr**-meh ah toh-dahs soos pah-**reh**-has ah-**sehr**-kah deh soo kohn-dee-**see-ohn**.
Use condoms all the time.	Use condones todo el tiempo. **Oo**-seh kohn-**doh**-nehs toh-doh ehl **tee-ehm**-poh.

Take your medicine, ___ pills
every ___ hours.

Tome su medicina,
___ pastillas cada ___ horas.
Toh-meh soo meh-dee-**see**-
nah, ___ pahs-**tee**-yhahs kah-
dah ___ **oh** rahs.

Return to the hospital if you
have . . .

Regrese al hospital si
tiene . . .
Re-**greh**-seh ahl **ohs**-pee-tahl
see **tee-eh**-neh . . .

___ fever

___ fiebre
fee-eh-breh

___ pain/swelling in the
joints

___ dolor/hinchazón en las
articulaciones
doh-**lohr**/een-chah-**sohn**
ehn lahs ahr-tee-koo-lah-
see-oh-nehs

___ skin rash

___ ronchas o manchas de la
piel
rohn-chahs oh **mahn**-
chahs deh lah pee-ehl

Testicular Pain / Swelling

Dolor / Hinchazón en el Testículo

Doh-**lohr** / een-chah-**sohn** ehn
ehl tehs-**tee-koo**-loh

How long has he (have you)
had the pain?

¿Por cuánto tiempo ha tenido
el dolor?
Pohr **kwahn**-toh **tee-ehm**-poh
ah teh-**nee**-doh ehl doh-**lohr?**

___ Hours

___ Days

Did the pain start suddenly?

Is the pain constant?

Does the pain come and go?

Does he (do you) have the pain now?

Did he (you) receive a hit in the scrotum?

Did he (you) fall?

Was he (were you) hit with a ball?

Was he (were you) kicked?

___ Horas
Oh-rahs

___ Días
Dee-ahs

¿Empezó el dolor de repente?
Ehm-peh-**soh** ehl doh-**lohr** deh reh-**pehn**-teh?

¿Es el dolor constante?
Ehs ehl doh-**lohr** kohns-**tahn**-teh?

¿Le va y viene el dolor?
Leh bah ee bee-eh-neh ehl doh-**lohr?**

¿Tiene el dolor ahora?
Tee-eh-neh ehl doh-**lohr** ah-**oh**-rah?

¿Recibió un golpe en el escroto?
Reh-see-**bee-oh** oon **gohl**-peh ehn ehl ehs-**kroh**-toh?

¿Se cayó?
Seh kah-**yoh?**

¿Recibió un golpe con una bola?
Reh-see-**bee-oh** oon **gohl**-peh kohn **oo**-nah boh-lah?

¿Lo patearon?
Loh pah-teh-**ah**-rohn?

Does he (do you) have swelling?	¿Tiene hinchazón? **Tee-eh**-neh een-chah-**sohn?**
Does he (do you) have vomiting?	¿Tiene vómito? **Tee-eh**-neh **boh**-mee-toh'?
Does he (do you) have abdominal pain?	¿Tiene dolor abdominal? **Tee-eh**-neh doh-**lohr** ab-doh-mee-**nahl?**
Does he (do you) have blood in his (your) urine?	¿Tiene sangre en la orina? **Tee-eh**-neh **sahn**-greh ehn lah oh-**ree**-nah?
Does he (do you) have penile discharge?	¿Tiene deshecho del pene? **Tee-eh**-neh dehs-**eh**-choh dehl **peh**-neh?

Common Terms for Scrotal Pain

I need to examine his / your testicles.	Necesito examinarle los testículos. Neh-seh-**see**-toh eg-sah-mee-**nahr**-leh lohs tehs-**tee-koo**-lohs.
I need a urine sample.	Necesito una muestra de orina. Neh-seh-**see**-toh **oo**-nah **mwehs**-trah deh oh-**ree**-nah.
He needs (you need) a blood test.	Necesita una prueba de sangre. Neh-seh-**see**-tah **oo**-nah **proo-eh**-bah deh **sahn**-greh.
He needs (you need) an ultrasound.	Necesita un ultrasonido. Neh-seh-**see**-tah oon **ool**-trah-soh-**nee**-doh.

He needs (you need) an operation (surgery).	Necesita una operación (cirugía). Neh-seh-**see**-tah **oo**-nah oh-peh-rah-**see-ohn** (see-roo-**hee**-ah).
He has (you have) testicular torsion.	Tiene el testículo torcido. **Tee-eh**-neh ehl tehs-**tee-koo**-loh tohr-**see**-doh.
He has (you have) an infection.	Tiene una infección. **Tee-eh**-neh **oo**-nah een-feg-**see-ohn.**
He has (you have) a hematoma.	Tiene un hematoma. **Tee-eh**-neh oon eh-mah-**toh**-mah.
He has (you have) a cyst.	Tiene un quiste. **Tee-eh**-neh oon **kees**-teh.

Discharge Instructions for Scrotal Pain

Return to the hospital if he has (you have) . . .	Regrese al hospital si tiene . . . Reh-**greh**-seh ahl **ohs**-pee-tahl see **tee-eh**-neh . . .
___ fever	___ fiebre **fee-eh**-breh
___ vomiting	___ vómito **boh**-mee-toh
___ worsening pain	___ peor dolor peh-**ohr** doh-**lohr**
___ more swelling	___ más hinchazón mahs een-chah-**sohn**

Give him the medicine every
___ hours.

Déle la medicina cada
___ horas.
Deh-leh lah meh-dee-**see**-nah
kah-dah ___ **oh**-rahs.

Go with the urologist on
___.

Vaya con el urólogo el día
___.
Bah-yah kohn ehl oo-**roh**-loh-
goh ehl **dee**-ah ___.

Psychiatry

Behavioral Change

Is there a change in his / her
behavior like . . . ?

___ fights too much with
friends or siblings

___ lies

___ steals

___ stays away from home
without permission

___ cries often without
reason

Does he / she usually obey
you on important matters?

Cambio de Comportamiento

Kahm-bee-oh deh kohm-pohr-
tah-mee-**ehn**-toh

¿Hay un cambio en su
comportamiento como . . . ?
Ah-ee oon **kahm**-bee-oh ehn
soo kohm-pohr-tah-mee-**ehn**-
toh, **koh**-moh . . . ?

___ pelea mucho con amigos
o hermanos
peh-**leh**-ah **moo**-choh
kohn ah-**mee**-gohs oh
ehr-**mah**-nohs

___ miente
mee-**ehn**-teh

___ roba
rho-bah

___ se queda fuera de casa
sin permiso
seh **keh**-dah **fweh**-rah
deh **kah**-sah seen pehr-
mee-soh

___ llora seguido sin razón
yoh-rah seh-**gee**-doh
seen rah-**sohn**

¿Usualmente le obedece en
asuntos importantes?
Oo-soo-ahl-**mehn**-teh leh oh-
beh-**deh**-seh ehn ah-**soon**-tohs
eem-pohr-**tahn**-tehs?

Is he / she always moving,
fidgeting, jumping around?

¿Se está moviendo, meneando,
brincando por todos lados?
Seh ehs-**tah** moh-bee-**ehn**-
doh, meh-neh-**ahn**-doh, breen-
kahn-doh pohr toh-dohs lah-
dohs?

Has he / she stopped playing
with friends and siblings?

¿Ha dejado de jugar con
amigos o hermanos?
Ah deh-**hah**-doh deh hoo-**gahr**
kohn ah **mee** gohs oh ehr
mah-nohs?

Does he / she urinate in bed?

¿Se orina en la cama?
Seh oh-**ree**-nah ehn lah **kah**-
mah?

How many nights per week?

¿Cuántas veces a la semana?
Kwahn-tahs **beh**-sehs ah lah
seh-**mah**-nah?

Is his / her behavior a
problem for you?

¿Es su comportamiento un
problema para usted?
Ehs soo kohm-pohr-tah-mee-
ehn-toh oon proh-**bleh**-mah
pah-rah oos-**tehd?**

Is his / her behavior a
problem for the teacher?

¿Es su comportamiento un
problema para el maestro?
Ehs soo kohm-pohr-tah-mee-
ehn-toh oon proh-**bleh**-mah
pah-rah ehl mah-**ehs**-troh?

What grade is he / she in
school?

¿En qué grado va en la
escuela?
Ehn **keh grah**-doh bah ehn lah
ehs-**kweh**-lah?

Is he / she failing any classes?

¿Está reprobando algunas
clases?
Ehs-**tah** reh-proh-**bahn**-doh
ahl-**goo**-nahs **klah**-sehs?

Does he / she have problems in school?

¿Tiene problemas en la escuela?
Tee-eh-neh proh-**bleh**-mahs ehn lah ehs-**kweh**-lah?

Has he / she been expelled or suspended from school lately?

¿Ha sido expulsado (a) o suspendido (a) de la escuela recientemente?
Ah see-doh egs-pool-**sah**-doh (dah) oh soos-pehn-**dee**-doh (dah) deh lah ehs-**kweh**-lah reh-see-**ehn**-teh-mehn-teh?

Does he / she cry or protest when he / she goes to school?

¿Llora o protesta cuando va a la escuela?
Yoh-rah oh proh-**tehs**-tah **kwahn**-doh bah ah lah ehs-**kweh**-lah?

Does he / she eat well?

¿Come bien?
Koh-meh bee-ehn?

Does he / she sleep well?

¿Duerme bien?
Dwehr-meh bee-ehn?

Does he / she stay alone in the room for a long time?

¿Se queda solo (a) en el cuarto por mucho tiempo?
Seh **keh**-dah soh-loh (lah) ehn ehl **kwahr**-toh pohr **moo**-choh **tee-ehm**-poh?

Is he / she losing weight?

¿Está perdiendo peso?
Ehs-**tah** pehr-dee-**ehn**-doh **peh**-soh?

Is he / she gaining weight?

¿Está aumentando de peso?
Ehs-**tah** ah-oo-mehn-**tahn**-doh deh **peh**-soh?

Does he / she seem sad or without energy?

¿Le parece a usted triste o sin energía?
Leh pah-**reh**-seh ah oos-**tehd trees**-teh oh seen eh-nehr-**hee**-ah?

Do you suspect that he / she uses drugs?

¿Sospecha usted que usa drogas?
Sohs-**peh**-chah oos-**tehd keh oo**-sah **droh** gahs?

Intentional Overdose

Sobredosis Intencional

Soh-breh-**doh**-sees een-tehn-see-oh-**nahl**

How many pills have you taken?

¿Cuántas pastillas ha tomado?
Kwahn-tahs pahs-**tee**-yahs ah toh-**mah**-doh?

What pills did you take?

¿Qué pastillas tomó?
Keh pahs-**tee**-yahs toh-**moh?**

___ Aspirin

___ Aspirina
Ahs-pee-**ree**-nah

___ Tylenol

___ Tylenol
Tay-leh-nohl

___ Ibuprofen

___ Ibuprofen
Ee-boo-proh-fehn

___ Antibiotic

___ Antibióticos
Ahn-tee-bee-**oh**-tee-kohs

___ Hypertension pills	___ Pastillas para la presión Pahs-**tee**-yahs pah-rah lah preh-**see-ohn**
___ Antidepressants	___ Pastillas para la depresión Pahs-**tee**-yahs pah-rah lah deh-preh-**see-ohn**
___ Dilantin	Dilantin Dee-lahn-teen
What time did you take the pills?	¿A qué hora tomó las pastillas? Ah **keh oh**-rah toh-**moh** lahs pahs-**tee**-yahs?
Did you bring the pill bottles with you?	¿Trajo los frascos de pastillas? **Trah**-hoh lohs **frahs**-kohs deh pahs-**tee**-yahs?
Did you drink alcohol?	¿Tomó alcohol? Toh-**moh** ahl-**kohl?**
Did you take the pills to kill yourself?	¿Tomó las pastillas para matarse? Toh-**moh** lahs pahs-**tee**-yahs pah-rah mah-**tahr**-seh?
Do you still want to kill yourself?	¿Todavía quiere matarse? Toh-dah-**bee**-ah kee-**eh**-reh mah-**tahr**-seh?
Have you tried to kill yourself before?	¿Ha tratado de matarse antes? Ah trah-**tah**-doh deh mah-**tahr**- seh **ahn**-tehs?
Do you suffer from depression?	¿Sufre de depresión? **Soo**-freh deh deh-preh-**see- ohn?**

Why did you want to kill yourself?	¿Por qué quizo matarse? Pohr **keh kee**-soh mah-**tahr**-seh?
___ Personal problems	___ Problemas personales Proh-**bleh**-mahs pehr-soh-**nah**-lehs
___ Problems at work	___ Problemas en el trabajo Proh-**bleh**-mahs ehn ehl trah **bah** hoh
___ Problems at school	___ Problemas en la escuela Proh-**bleh**-mahs ehn lah ehs-**kweh**-lah
___ Problems with parents	___ Problemas con los padres Proh-**bleh**-mahs kohn lohs **pah**-drehs
___ Problems with girlfriend / boyfriend	___ Problemas con la novia / el novio Proh-**bleh**-mahs kohn lah **noh**-bee-ah / ehl **noh**-bee-oh
Have you taken drugs?	¿Ha tomado drogas? Ah toh-**mah**-doh **droh**-gahs
___ Marihuana	___ Marijuana Mah-ree-**hwah**-nah
___ Cocaine	___ Cocaína Koh-kah-**ee**-nah
___ Heroin	___ Heroína Eh-roh-**ee**-nah
Do you have abdominal pain?	¿Tiene dolor abdominal? **Tee-eh**-neh doh-**lohr** ab-doh-mee-**nahl?**

Do you have nausea or vomiting?

¿Tiene náusea o vómito?
Tee-eh-neh **nah**-oo-seh-ah oh **boh**-mee-toh?

Have you vomited since you took the pills?

¿Ha vomitado desde que tomó las pastillas?
Ah boh-mee-**tah**-doh dehs-deh **keh** toh-**moh** lahs pahs-**tee**-yahs?

Do you have dizziness?

¿Tiene mareos?
Tee-eh-neh mah-**reh**-ohs?

Do you have chest pain?

¿Tiene dolor de pecho?
Tee-eh-neh doh-**lohr** deh **peh**-choh?

Common Terms for Intentional Overdose

I need to put a tube through your mouth to empty your stomach.

Necesito ponerle un tubo por la boca para vaciarle el estómago.
Neh-seh-**see**-toh poh-**nehr**-leh oon **too**-boh pohr lah **boh**-kah pah-rah bah-see-**ahr**-leh ehl ehs-**toh**-mah-goh.

You need a nasogastric tube.

Necesita una sonda nasogástrica.
Neh-seh-**see**-tah **oo**-nah **sohn**-dah nah-soh-**gahs**-tree-kah.

You need to take medicine to neutralize the pills you took.

Necesita tomar medicina para neutralizar las pastillas que tomó.
Neh-seh-**see**-tah toh-**mahr** meh-dee-**see**-nah pah-rah neh-oo-trah-lee-**sahr** lahs pahs-**tee**-yahs **keh** toh-**moh.**

You need to see a psychiatrist.

Necesita ver a un psiquiatra.
Neh-seh-**see**-tah behr ah oon
see-kee-**ah**-trah.

We need to admit you.

Necesitamos internarlo (a).
Neh-seh-see-**tah**-mohs **een**-
tehr-**nahr**-loh (lah).

Discharge Instructions for Intentional Overdose

Return to the hospital if . . .

Regrese al hospital si . . .
Reh-**greh**-seh ahl **ohs**-pee-tahl
see . . .

a. you have abdominal pain
and / or vomiting.

a. tiene dolor abdominal o
vómito
tee-**eh**-neh doh-**lohr** ab-
doh-mee-**nahl** oh **boh**-mee-
toh

b. feel like hurting yourself or
others

b. siente que va a lastimarse o
va a lastimar a otros
see-**ehn**-teh **keh** bah ah
lahs-tee-**mahr**-seh oh bah
ah lahs-tee-**mahr** ah oh-
trohs

c. you have dizziness

c. tiene mareos
Tee-**eh**-neh mah-**reh**-ohs

Depression and Suicidal Ideation

Depresión e Ideas Suicidas

Deh-preh-**see-ohn** eh ee-**deh**-
ahs soo-ee-**see**-dahs

Is he / she depressed?

¿Esta deprimido (a)?
Ehs-**tah** deh-pree-**mee**-doh
(dah)?

For how long has he / she had depression?

¿Por cuánto tiempo ha tenido depresión?
Pohr **kwahn**-toh **tee-ehm**-poh
ah teh-**nee**-doh deh-preh-**see-ohn?**

Does he / she have trouble sleeping?

¿Tiene dificultades para dormir?
Tee-eh-neh dee-fee-kool-**tah**-dehs pah-rah dohr-**meer?**

How many hours a day does he / she sleep?

¿Cuántas horas duerme al día?
Kwahn-tahs **oh**-rahs **dwehr**-meh ahl **dee**-ah?

Does he / she wake up at dawn?

¿Se levanta en la madrugada?
Seh leh-**bahn**-tah ehn lah mah-droo-**gah**-dah?

Does he / she have a lack of appetite?

¿Tiene falta de apetito?
Tee-eh-neh fahl-tah deh ah-peh-**tee**-toh?

Does he / she cry for any reason?

¿Llora por cualquier cosa?
Yoh-rah pohr kwahl-kee-**ehr koh**-sah?

Does he / she feel without value?

¿Siente que no tiene valor?
See-ehn-teh keh noh **tee-eh**-neh bah-**lohr?**

Does he / she hear voices?

¿Oye voces?
Oh-yeh **boh**-sehs?

When did he / she start hearing voices?

¿Cuándo empezó a oir voces?
Kwahn-doh ehm-peh-**soh** ah oh-**eer boh**-sehs?

Do the voices tell him / her to hurt or kill himself / herself?

¿Le dicen las voces que se lastime o que se suicide?
Leh **dee**-sehn lahs **boh**-sehs **keh** seh lahs-**tee**-meh oh **keh** seh soo-ee-**see**-deh?

Do the voices tell him / her to hurt other people?

¿Le dicen las voces que lastime a otras personas?
Leh **dee**-sehn lahs **boh**-sehs **keh** lahs-**tee**-meh ah oh-trahs pehr-**son**-nahs?

Has he / she ever tried to kill himself / herself before?

¿Ha tratado de matarse antes?
Ah trah-**tah**-doh deh mah-**tahr**-seh **ahn**-tehs?

When?

¿Cuándo?
Kwahn-doh?

___ Month

___ Mes
Mehs

___ Year

___ Año
Ah-nyoh

How many times has he / she tried to kill himself / herself?

¿Cuántas veces ha intentado matarse?
Kwahn-tahs **beh**-sehs ah een-tehn-**tah**-doh mah-**tahr**-seh?

How did he / she try to kill himself / herself?

¿Cómo trató de matarse?
Koh-moh trah-**toh** deh mah-**tahr**-seh?

___ With pills

___ Con pastillas
Kohn pahs-**tee**-yahs

___ With a knife

___ Con un cuchillo
Kohn oon koo-**chee**-yoh

___ With a gun

___ Con una pistola
Kohn **oo**-nah pees-**toh**-lah

___ Jumping from a high place

___ Saltando de un lugar alto
Sahl-**tahn**-doh deh oon loo-**gahr ahl**-toh

___ Hanging

___ Ahorcándose
Ah-ohr-**kahn**-dose

Does he / she still want to kill himself / herself?

¿Todavía quiere matarse?
Toh-dah-**bee**-ah kee-**eh**-reh mah-**tahr**-seh?

Does he / she think that the TV / radio only speaks to him / her?

¿Cree que la televisíon / radio solamente le habla a él / ella?
Kreh-eh **keh** lah teh-leh-bee-**see-ohn** / **rah**-dee-oh soh-lah-**mehn**-teh leh **ah**-blah ah ehl / eh-yah?

Does he / she think that someone is following him / her?

¿Cree que alguién le persigue?
Kreh-eh **keh** ahl-gee-**ehn** leh pehr-**see**-geh?

Does he / she think that people are talking behind his / her back?

¿Cree que la gente habla de él / ella detrás de su espalda?
Kreh-eh **keh** lah **gehn**-teh **ah**-blah deh ehl / eh-yah deh-**trahs** deh soo ehs-**pahl**-dah?

Has he / she seen a psychiatrist?

¿Ha visto a un psiquiatra?
Ah **bees**-toh ah oon see-kee-**ah**-trah?

Has he / she been admitted to a psychiatric hospital?

¿Lo (la) han internado (a) en un hospital psiquiátrico?
Loh (lah) ahn een-tehr-**nah**-doh (dah) ehn oon **ohs**-pee-tahl see-kee-**ah**-tree-koh?

Does he / she take medication for depression?

¿Está tomando medicina para la depresión?
Ehs-**tah** toh-**mahn**-doh meh-dee-**see**-nah pah-rah lah deh-preh-**see-ohn?**

Which medicine?

¿Cuál medicina?
Kwahl meh-dee-**see**-nah?

___ Haldol

___ Haldol
Hal-dohl

___ Elavil

___ Elavil
Eh-lah-beel

___ Prolixin

___ Prolixin
Proh-leeks-seen

___ Thorazine

___ Thorazine
Toh-rah-seen

___ Zoloft

___ Zoloft
Soh-lofht

___ Paxil

___ Paxil
Pak-seel

___ Valium

___ Valium
Bah-lee-uhm

Does he / she drink alcohol?

¿Toma alcohol?
Toh-mah ahl-**kohl?**

When was the last time he / she drank?

¿Cuándo fué la última vez que tomó?
Kwahn-doh **fweh** lah **ool**-tee-mah behs **keh** toh-**moh?**

Does he / she use drugs like . . . ?

¿Usa drogas como . . . ?
Oo-sah **droh**-gahs **koh**-moh . . . ?

___ marihuana

___ marijuana
mah-ree-**hwah**-nah

___ cocaine

___ cocaína
koh-kah-**ee**-nah

___ heroin (inhaled or IV)

___ heroína (inhalada o intravenosa)
eh-roh-**ee**-nah (een-ah-**lah**-dah oh een-trah-beh-**noh**-sah)

___ mushrooms

___ hongos
ohn-gohs

___ crack cocaine

___ rocas de cocaína (crack)
roh-kahs de koh-kah-**ee**-nah

Common Terms for Depression and Suicidal Ideation

He / she needs to see a psychiatrist.

Él / ella necesita ver a un psiquiatra.
Ehl / eh-yah neh-seh-**see**-tah behr ah oon see-kee-**ah**-trah.

We need to restrain him / her for his / her protection

Necesitamos atarlo (la) para su protección.
Neh-seh-see-**tah**-mohs ah-**tahr**-loh (lah) pah-rah soo proh-tek-**see-ohn.**

We are going to send him / her to a psychiatric hospital.

Vamos a mandarlo (la) a un hospital psiquiátrico.
Bah-mohs ah mahn-**dahr**-loh (lah) ah oon **ohs**-pee-tahl see-kee-**ah**-tree-koh.

We are going to give him /
her pills for the depression.

Vamos a darle pastillas para la
depresión.
Bah-mohs ah dahr-leh pahs-
tee-yhahs pah-rah lah deh-
preh-**see-ohn.**

Discharge Instructions for Depression and Suicidal Ideation

Return to the hospital if . . .

Regrese al hospital si . . .
Reh-**greh**-seh ahl **ohs**-pee-tahl
see . . .

___ he / she feels depressed

___ él / ella se siente
deprimido (a)
ehl / eh-yah seh **see-
ehn**-teh deh-pree-**mee**-
doh (ah)

___ he / she thinks about
hurting himself / herself

___ piensa que se va a
lastimar
pee-**ehn**-sah **keh** seh
bah ah lahs-tee-**mahr**

___ he / she thinks about
hurting others

___ piensa que va a lastimar
a otros
pee-**ehn**-sah **keh** bah ah
lahs-tee-**mahr** ah oh-
trohs

Take the medicine as
indicated.

Tome la medicina como le
indicaron.
Toh-meh lah meh-dee-**see**-nah
koh-moh leh een-dee-**kah**-
rohn.

See the psychiatrist soon.

Vea al psiquiatra pronto.
Beh-ah ahl see-kee-**ah**-trah
prohn-toh.

Miscellaneous

Accidental Overdose

Sobredosis Accidental

Soh-breh-**doh**-sees ag-see-dehn-**tahl**

When did he / she take the pills?	¿Cuándo tomó las pastillas? **Kwahn**-doh toh-**moh** lahs pahs-**tee**-yahs?
How many pills did he / she take?	¿Cuántas pastillas tomó? **Kwahn**-tahs pahs-**tee**-yahs toh-**moh?**
What pills did he / she take?	¿Qué pastillas tomó? **Keh** pahs-**tee**-yahs toh-**moh?**

___ Aspirin

___ Aspirina
Ahs-pee-**ree**-nah

___ Tylenol

___ Tylenol
Tay-leh-nohl

___ Ibuprofen

___ Ibuprofen
Ee-boo-proh-fehn

___ Antibiotics

___ Antibióticos
Ahn-tee-bee-**oh**-tee-kohs

___ High blood pressure pills

___ Pastillas para la alta presión
Pahs-**tee**-yahs pah-rah lah **ahl**-tah preh-**see-ohn**

___ Heart pills

___ Pastillas para el corazón
Pahs-**tee**-yahs pah-rah ehl koh-rah-**sohn**

___ Diabetes pills

___ Pastillas para la diabetes
Pahs-**tee**-yahs pah-rah
lah dee-ah-**beh**-tehs

___ Antidepressant pills

___ Pastillas para la
depresión
Pahs-**tee**-yahs pah-rah
lah deh-preh-**see-ohn**

Did you bring the pill bottles
with you?

¿Trajo con usted los frascos de
las pastillas?
Trah-ho kohn oos-**tehd** lohs
frahs-kohs deh lahs pash-**tee**-
yahs?

Did he / she vomit after
taking the pills?

¿Vomitó después de tomar las
pastillas?
Boh-mee-**toh** dehs-**pwehs** deh
toh-**mahr** lahs pahs-**tee**-yahs?

Have you seen any pills in the
vomit?

¿Ha visto pastillas en el
vómito?
Ah **bees**-toh pahs-**tee**-yahs
ehn ehl **boh**-mee-toh?

Did he / she spit the pills?

¿Escupió las pastillas?
Ehs-koo-**pee-oh** lahs pahs-**tee**-
yahs?

Did he / she chew the pills?

¿Masticó las pastillas?
Mahs-tee-**koh** lahs pahs-**tee**-
yahs?

Did he / she drink / eat
anything since the ingestion?

¿Tomó o comió algo después
de la ingestion?
Toh-**moh** oh koh-mee-**oh** ahl-
goh dehs-**pwehs** deh lah een-
hes-tee-**ohn?**

Does he / she have a fever?	¿Tiene fiebre? **Tee-eh**-neh **fee-eh**-breh?
Does he / she have abdominal pain?	¿Tiene dolor abdominal? **Tee-eh**-neh doh-**lohr** ab-doh-mee-**nahl?**
Has he / she been acting normal since the ingestion?	¿Ha estado actuando normal desde la ingestion? Ah ehs-**tah**-doh ahk-too-**ahn**-doh nohr-**mahl** dehs-deh lah een-hes-tee-**ohn?**
Is he / she more sleepy than normal?	¿Tiene más sueño de lo normal? **Tee-eh**-neh mahs soo-**eh**-nyoh deh loh nohr-**mahl?**
Is he / she walking fine?	¿Camina bien? Kah-**mee**-nah bee-ehn?
Is he / she speaking well?	¿Habla bien? **Ah**-blah bee-ehn?
Does he / she have problems breathing?	¿Tiene problemas para respirar? **Tee-eh**-neh proh-**bleh**-mahs pah-rah rehs-pee-**rahr?**

Common Terms During the Exam for Accidental Overdose

| He / she needs blood tests. | Él / ella necesita análisis de sangre.
Ehl / eh-yah neh-seh-**see**-tah ah-**nah**-lee-sees deh **sahn**-greh. |

He / she needs a nasogastric tube.

Él / ella necesita un tubo nasogástrico.
Ehl / eh-yah neh-seh-**see**-tah oon **too**-boh nah-soh-**gas**-tree-koh.

We need to empty his / her stomach.

Necesitamos vaciarle el estómago.
Neh-seh-see-**tah**-mohs bah-see-**ahr**-leh ehl ehs-**toh**-mah-ɡnh

He / she needs medicine to neutralize the pills.

Él / ella necesita medicina para neutralizar las pastillas.
Ehl / eh-yah neh-seh-**see**-tah meh-dee-**see**-nah pah-rah nee-oo-trah-lee-**sahr** lahs pahs-**tee**-yahs.

We need to admit him / her.

Necesitamos internarlo (la).
Neh-seh-see-**tah**-mohs **een**-tehr-**nahr**-loh (lah).

The ingestion was minimal.

La ingestion fué mínima.
Lah een-hes-tee-**ohn fweh mee**-nee-mah.

Discharge Instructions for Accidental Overdose

Return to the hospital if he / she has . . .

Regrese al hospital si él / ella tiene . . .
Reh-**greh**-seh ahl **ohs**-pee-tahl see ehl / eh-yah **tee-eh**-neh . . .

___ fever

___ fiebre
fee-eh-breh

___ problems breathing

___ problemas para respirar
proh-**bleh**-mahs pah-rah rehs-pee-**rahr**

___ behavior change

___ cambio en su
comportamiento
kahm-bee-oh ehn soo
kohm-pohr-tah-mee-**ehn**-
toh

___ excessive sleepiness or
drowsiness

___ sueño excessivo
soo-**eh**-nyoh eg-seh-**see**-
boh

Keep all medications out of
the child's reach.

Mantenga toda la medicina
fuera del alcance del niño (a).
Mahn-**tehn**-gah toh-dah lah
meh-dee-**see**-nah **fweh**-rah
dehl ahl-**kahn**-seh dehl **nee**-
nyoh (nyah).

Bites (Human, Animal, Insect)

Mordidas

Mohr-**dee**-dahs

When was he / she bitten?

¿Cuándo lo / la mordieron?
Kwahn-doh loh / lah mohr-
dee-**eh**-rohn?

Was he / she bitten by
another person?

¿Fué mordido (a) por otra
persona?
Fweh mohr-**dee**-doh (ah) pohr
oh-trah pehr-**soh**-nah?

Was he / she bitten by an
animal?

¿Fué mordido (a) por un
animal?
Fweh mohr-**dee**-doh (ah) pohr
oon ah-nee-**mahl?**

What animal bit him / her?	¿Qué animal lo / la mordió? **Keh** ah-nee-**mahl** loh / lah mohr-dee-**oh?**
___ A dog	___ Un perro Oon **peh**-rho
___ A cat	___ Un gato Oon **gah**-toh
___ A squirrel	___ Una ardilla **Oo**-nah ahr-**dee**-yah
___ A mouse or rat	___ Un ratón o rata Oon rah-**tohn** oh **rah**-tah
Was he / she stung by an insect?	¿Le picó un insecto? Leh pee-**koh** oon een-**sek**-toh?
___ A mosquito	___ Un mosquito Oon mohs-**kee**-toh
___ A bee	___ Una abeja **Oo**-nah ah-**beh**-hah
___ A spider	___ Una araña **Oo**-nah ah-**rah**-nyah
Does he / she have a laceration?	¿Tiene una laceración / cortada? **Tee-eh**-neh **oo**-nah lah-seh-rah-**see-ohn** / kohr-**tah**-dah?
Is there discharge from the wound?	¿Hay deshecho de la herida? Ay dehs-**eh**-choh deh lah eh-**ree**-dah?
Is it red around the wound?	¿Tiene rojo alrededor de la herida? **Tee-eh**-neh **roh**-ho ahl-reh-deh-**dohr** deh lah eh-**ree**-dah?

Does he / she have fever?

¿Tiene fiebre?
Tee-eh-neh **fee-eh**-breh?

Is the wound swollen?

¿Está hinchada la herida?
Ehs-**tah** een-**chah**-dah lah eh-**ree**-dah?

Do you know the dog (cat) that bit him / her?

¿Usted conoce el perro (gato) que lo / la mordió?
Oos-**tehd** koh-**noh**-seh ehl **peh**-rho (**gah**-toh) **keh** loh / lah mohr-dee-**oh?**

Do you know if the animal is vaccinated?

¿Sabe usted si el animal está vacunado?
Sah-beh oos-**tehd** see ehl ah-nee-**mahl** ehs-**tah** bah-koo-**nah**-doh?

Did you report the attack to the police?

¿Reportó el ataque a la policía?
Reh-pohr-**toh** ehl ah-**tah**-keh ah lah poh-lee-**see**-ah?

Is the child up to date with the vaccines?

¿Está al corriente el niño / la niña con las vacunas?
Ehs-**tah** ahl koh-ree-**ehn**-teh ehl **nee**-nyoh / lah **nee**-nyah kohn lahs bah-**koo**-nahs?

Is he / she allergic to penicillin?

¿Es alérgico (a) a la penicilina?
Ehs ah-**lehr**-hee-koh ah lah peh-nee-see-**lee**-nah?

Common Terms for Bites

We have to clean the wound.

Necesitamos limpiar la herida.
Neh-seh-see-**tah**-mohs leem-pee-**ahr** lah eh-**ree**-dah.

He / she needs sutures.

Él / ella necesita puntadas / suturas.
Ehl / eh-yah neh-seh-**see**-tah poon-**tah**-dahs / soo-**too**-rahs.

He / she needs a tetanus vaccine.

Él / ella necesita una vacuna del tétano.
Ehl / eh-yah neh-seh-**see**-tah **oo**-nah bah-**koo**-nah dehl **teh**-tah-noh.

He / she needs a rabies vaccine.

Él / ella necesita una vacuna para la rabia.
Ehl / eh-yah neh-seh-**see**-tah **oo**-nah bah-**koo**-nah pah-rah lah **rha**-bee-ah.

He / she does not need a rabies vaccine.

Él / ella no necesita una vacuna para la rabia.
Ehl / eh-yah no neh-seh-**see**-tah **oo**-nah bah-**koo**-nah pah-rah lah **rha**-bee-ah.

He / she needs antibiotics.

Él / ella necesita antibióticos.
Ehl / eh-yah neh-seh-**see**-tah ahn-tee-bee-**oh**-tee-kohs.

I am not going to suture the wound so it does not become infected.

No voy a ponerle puntadas para que no se le infecte la herida.
Noh boy ah poh-**nehr**-leh poon-**tah**-dahs pah-rah **keh** noh seh leh een-**fek**-teh lah eh-**ree**-dah.

Discharge Instructions for Bites

Keep the wound clean and dry.

Mantenga la herida limpia y seca.
Mahn-**tehn**-gah lah eh-**ree**-dah **leem**-pee-ah ee **seh**-kah.

Return to the hospital if he / she has . . .

Regrese al hospital si él / ella tiene . . .
Reh-**greh**-seh ahl **ohs**-pee-tahl see ehl / eh-yah **tee-eh**-neh . . .

___ redness around the wound

___ rojo alrededor de la herida
roh-ho ahl-reh-deh-**dohr** deh lah eh-**ree**-dah

___ pus from the wound

___ pus de la herida
poos deh lah eh-**ree**-dah

___ fever

___ fiebre
fee-eh-breh

___ more pain or swelling

___ más dolor o hinchazón
mahs doh-**lohr** oh een-chah-**sohn**

Give him / her Tylenol (Advil) for the pain every ___ hours.

Déle Tylenol (Advil) para el dolor cada ___ horas.
Deh-leh Tay-leh-nohl / Ad-beel pah-rah ehl doh-**lohr** kah-dah ___ **oh**-rahs.

Give him / her antibiotics every ___ hours.

Déle antibióticos cada ___ horas.
Deh-leh ahn-tee-bee-**oh**-tee-kohs kah-dah ___ **oh**-rahs.

Burns

Quemaduras

Keh-mah-**doo**-rahs

What was he / she burned with?

¿Con qué se quemó?
Kohn **keh** seh keh-**moh?**

___ Hot water

___ Agua caliente
Ah-gwah kah-lee-**ehn**-
teh

___ Hot oil

___ Aceite caliente
Ah-**say**-teh kah-lee-**ehn**-
teh

___ House radiator

___ Un radiador de casa
Oon rah-dee-ah-**dohr**
deh **kah**-sah

___ An iron

___ Una plancha
Oo-nah **plahn**-chah

___ The stove

___ La estufa
Lah ehs-**too**-fah

___ Fire

___ Fuego / lumbre
Fweh-goh / **loom**-breh

___ A cigarette

___ Un cigarrillo
Oon see-gah-**rhee**-yoh

When was he / she burnt?

¿Cuándo se quemó?
Kwahn-doh seh keh-**moh?**

___ Hours ago

Hace ___ horas
Ah-seh   **oh**-rahs

___ days ago

___ días
dee-ahs

Does he / she have fever?

¿Tiene fiebre?
Tee-eh-neh **fee-eh**-breh?

Does he / she have pus
(discharge) from the burn?

¿Tiene pus (deshecho) de la
quemadura?
Tee-eh-neh poos (dehs-**eh**-
choh) deh lah keh-mah-**doo**-
rah?

Does he / she have pain?	¿Tiene dolor? **Tee-eh**-neh doh-**lohr?**
When was the last time he / she received a tetanus vaccine?	¿Cuándo fué la última vez que recibió una vacuna del tétano? **Kwahn**-doh **fweh** lah **ool**-tee-mah behs **keh** reh-see-**bee-oh** **oo**-nah bah-**koo**-nah dehl **teh**-tah-noh?
Does he / she have allergies?	¿Tiene alérgias? **Tee-eh**-neh ah-**lehr**-hee-ahs?

Common Terms for Burns

I need to clean the burn.	Necesito limpiarle la quemadura. Neh-seh-**see**-toh leem-pee-**ahr**-leh lah keh-mah-**doo**-rah.
He / she needs a special cream for the burn.	Él / ella necesita una crema especial para la quemadura. Ehl / eh-yah neh-seh-**see**-tah **oo**-nah **kreh**-mah ehs-peh-see-**ahl** pah-rah lah keh-mah-**doo**-rah.
He / she needs to see a burn specialist.	Él / ella necesita ver a un especialista de quemaduras. Ehl / eh-yah neh-seh-**see**-tah behr ah oon ehs-**peh-see**-ah-lees-tah deh keh-mah-**doo**-rahs.
He / she has an infection.	Tiene una infección. **Tee-eh**-neh **oo**-nah een-feg-**see-ohn.**
He / she needs antibiotics.	Necesita antibióticos. Neh-seh-**see**-tah ahn-tee-bee-**oh**-tee-kohs.

He / she needs to be admitted.

Necesitamos admitirlo (la).
Neh-seh-see-**tah**-mohs ahd-mee-**teer**-loh (lah).

Discharge Instructions for Burns

Change his / her dressing daily and apply Silvadene.

Cambie sus vendajes / gazas diariamente y aplique Silvadene.
Kahm-bee soos behn-**dah**-hehs / **gah**-sahs dee-**ah**-riah-mehn-teh ee ah-**plee**-keh Seel-bah-deen.

Return to the hospital if he / she has . . .

Regrese al hospital si él / ella tiene . . .
Reh-**greh**-seh ahl **ohs**-pee-tahl see ehl / eh-yah **tee-eh**-neh . . .

___ redness around the burn

___ rojo alrededor de la quemadura
roh-ho ahl-reh-deh-**dohr** deh lah keh-mah-**doo**-rah

___ pus from the burn

___ pus de la quemadura
poos deh lah keh-mah-**doo**-rah

___ fever

___ fiebre
fee-eh-breh

Give him / her Tylenol / Advil for the pain every ___ hours.

Déle Tylenol / Advil para el dolor cada ___ horas.
Deh-leh Tay-leh-nohl / Ad-beel pah-rah ehl doh-**lohr** kah-dah ___ **oh**-rahs.

Smoke Inhalation

Inhalación de Humo
Een-ah-lah-**see-ohn** deh **oo**-moh

How long was he / she in the smoke?

¿Cuánto tiempo estuvo en el humo?
Kwahn-toh **tee-ehm**-poh ehs-**too**-boh ehn ehl **oo**-moh?

Was there ventilation in the room?

¿Había ventilación en el cuarto?
Ah-**bee**-ah behn-tee-lah-**see-ohn** ehn ehl **kwarh**-toh?

Does he / she feel short of breath?

¿Siente falta de aire?
See-ehn-teh fahl-tah deh **ay**-reh?

Does he / she have a cough?

¿Tiene tos?
Tee-eh-neh tohs?

Does he / she have phlegm?

¿Tiene flema?
Tee-eh-neh **fleh**-mah?

Have you noticed black phlegm?

¿Ha notado flema negra?
Ah noh-**tah**-doh **fleh**-mah **neh**-grah?

Does he / she have wheezing?

¿Tiene silbidos en el pecho?
Tee-eh-neh seel-**bee**-dohs ehn ehl **peh**-choh?

Does he / she have pain in the throat?

¿Tiene dolor en la garganta?
Tee-eh-neh doh-**lohr** ehn lah gahr-**gahn**-tah?

Is he / she hoarse?

¿Está ronco (a)?
Ehs-**tah rhon**-koh (kah)?

Does his / her chest hurt?

¿Le duele el pecho?
Leh **dweh**-leh ehl **peh**-choh?

Does he / she feel dizzy?

¿Se siente mareado (a)?
Seh **see-ehn**-teh mah-reh-**ah**-
doh (dah)?

Does he / she have a
headache?

¿Tiene dolor de cabeza?
Tee-eh-neh doh-**lohr** deh kah-
beh-sah?

Does he / she have nausea or
vomiting?

¿Tiene náusca o vómito?
Tee-eh-neh **nah**-oo-seh-ah oh
boh-mee-toh?

Common Terms for Smoke Inhalation

I need to do an arterial blood
test.

Necesito hacerle una prueba
de sangre arterial.
Neh-seh-**see**-toh ah-**sehr**-leh
oo-nah **proo-eh**-bah deh
sahn-greh ahr-teh-ree-**ahl.**

He / she needs an X-ray.

Él / ella necesita rayos X.
Ehl / eh-yah neh-seh-**see**-tah
rah-yohs **eh**-keys.

We need to intubate him /
her.

Necesitamos intubarlo (a).
Neh-seh-see-**tah**-mohs een-
too-**bahr**-loh (ah).

He / she needs oxygen.

Él / ella necesita oxígeno.
Ehl / eh-yah neh-seh-**see**-tah
ohg-**see**-heh-noh.

Discharge Instructions for Smoke Inhalation

Return to the hospital if he / she has . . .

Regrese al hospital si él / ella tiene . . .
Reh-**greh**-seh ahl **ohs**-pee-tahl see ehl / eh-yah **tee-eh**-neh . . .

— headache or dizziness

— dolor de cabeza o mareos
doh-**lohr** deh kah-**beh**-sah oh mah-**reh**-ohs

— shortness of breath

— falta de aire
fahl-tah deh ay-reh

— wheezing

— silbidos en el pecho
seel-**bee**-dohs ehn ehl **peh**-choh

— choking sensation

— sensación de estar sofocado
sehn-sah-**see-ohn** deh ehs-**tahr** soh-foh-**kah**-doh

Lead Screening / Toxicity

Intoxicación del Plomo

Een-tog-see-kah-**see-ohn** dehl **ploh**-moh

Does the child eat dirt or paint from the wall?

¿El niño / la niña come tierra o pintura de la pared?
Ehl **nee**-nyoh / lah **nee**-nyah **koh**-meh **tee-eh**-rha oh peen-**too**-rah deh lah pah-**rehd?**

Is there peeling paint at your home?

¿Hay pintura que se esté pelando en su casa?
Ay peen-**too**-rah **keh** seh ehs-**teh** peh-**lahn**-doh ehn soo **kah**-sah?

Do you know if there is lead paint in your home?

¿Sabe si hay pintura con plomo en su casa?
Sah-beh see ay peen-**too**-rah kohn **ploh**-moh ehn soo **kah**-sah?

Does the child live in a home or building (school or daycare) built before 1960?

¿Vive el niño / la niña en una casa o edificio (escuela o guardería) construída antes de 1960?
Bee-beh ehl **nee**-nyoh / lah **nee**-nyah ehn **oo**-nah **kah**-sah oh eh-dee-**fee**-see-oh (ehs-**kweh**-lah oh gwahr-deh-**ree**-ah) kohns-troo-**ee**-dah **ahn**-tehs deh 1960?

Has the child ever lived in a home or building (school or daycare) built before 1960?

¿Ha vivido el niño / la niña en una casa o edificio (escuela o guardería) construída antes de 1960?
Ah bee-**bee**-doh ehl **nee**-nyoh / lah **nee**-nyah ehn **oo**-nah **kah**-sah oh eh-dee-**fee**-see-oh (ehs-**kweh**-lah oh gwahr-deh-**ree**-ah) kohns-troo-**ee**-dah **ahn**-tehs deh 1960?

Does the child regularly visit a home or building (school or daycare) built before 1960?

¿Visita el niño / la niña regularmente una casa o edificio (escuela o guardería) construída antes de 1960?
Bee-**see**-tah ehl **nee**-nyoh / lah **nee**-nyah reh-goo-lahr-**mehn**-teh **oo**-nah **kah**-sah oh eh-dee-**fee**-see-oh (ehs-**kweh**-lah oh gwahr-deh-**ree**-ah) kohns-troo-**ee**-dah **ahn**-tehs deh 1960?

Does the child live in a home or building built before 1960 that has recently or is currently under renovation or remodeling?

¿Vive el niño / la niña en una casa o edificio construída antes de 1960 que recientemente ha sido o está siendo renovada o remodelada?
Bee-beh ehl **nee**-nyoh lah **nee**-nyah ehn **oo**-nah **kah**-sah oh eh-dee-**fee**-see-oh kohns-troo-**ee**-dah **ahn**-tehs deh 1960 **keh** reh-see-**ehn**-teh-mehn-teh ah see-doh oh ehs-**tah** see-**ehn**-doh rhe-noh-**bah**-dah oh rhe-moh-deh-**lah**-dah?

Does the child regularly visit a home or building built before 1960 that has recently or is currently under renovation or remodeling?

¿Visita el niño / la niña regularmente una casa o edificio construída antes de 1960 que recientemente ha sido o está siendo renovada o remodelada?
Bee-**see**-tah ehl **nee**-nyoh / lah **nee**-nyah reh-goo-lahr-**mehn**-teh **oo**-nah **kah**-sah oh eh-dee-**fee**-see-oh kohns-troo-**ee**-dah **ahn**-tehs deh 1960 **keh** reh-see-**ehn**-teh-mehn-teh ah see-doh oh ehs-**tah** see-**ehn**-doh rhe-noh-**bah**-dah oh rhe-moh-deh-**lah**-dah?

Does the child live with a person whose occupation or hobby involves exposure to lead, such as . . . ?

¿Vive el niño / la niña con una persona cuya ocupación o hobby tenga que ver con el plomo, como . . . ?
Bee beh chl **nee** nyoh / lah **nee**-nyah kohn **oo**-nah pehr-**soh**-nah **koo**-yah oh-koo-pah-**see-ohn** oh hob-bee **tehn**-gah **keh** behr kohn ehl **ploh**-moh, **koh**-mo . . . ?

___ construction

___ construcción
kohns-trook-**see-ohn**

___ welding

___ soldadura
sohl-dah-**doo**-rah

___ pottery

___ cerámica
seh-**rah**-mee-kah

Do you live near an industrial area or factory?

¿Vive usted cerca de una área industrial o fábrica?
Bee-beh oos-**tehd sehr**-kah deh **oo**-nah **ah**-reh-ah een-doos-tree-**ahl** oh **fah**-bree-kah?

What type of factory?

¿Qué tipo de fábrica?
Keh tee-poh deh **fah**-bree-kah?

___ Construction

___ Construcción
Kohns-trook-**see-ohn**

___ Steel

___ Acero
Ah-**seh**-roh

___ Paint

___ Pintura
Peen-**too**-rah

___ Chemical

___ De química
Deh **kee**-mee-kah

Does the child receive or has ever received herbal medicines or home remedies?

¿Recibe el niño / la niña o alguna vez ha recibido medicina a base de hierbas o remedios caseros?
Reh-**see**-beh ehl **nee**-nyoh / lah **nee**-nyah oh ahl-**goo**-nah behs ah reh-see-**bee**-doh meh-dee-**see**-nah ah bah-seh deh **yehr**-bahs oh reh-**meh**-dee-ohs kah-**seh**-rohs?

Has your child been tested for lead poisoning?

¿Ha tenido el examen del plomo su niño (a)?
Ah teh-**nee**-doh ehl eg-**sah**-mehn dehl **ploh**-moh soo **nee**-nyoh (ah)

If yes, when?

Si fué asi, cuándo?
See **fweh** ah-**see, kwahn**-doh?

Do you know the results?

¿Sabe los resultados?
Sah-beh lohs reh-sool-**tah**-dohs?

Does he / she complain of abdominal pain?

¿Se queja de dolor abdominal?
Seh **keh**-hah deh doh-**lohr** ab-doh-mee-**nahl?**

Is he / she constipated?

¿Está estreñido (a)?
Ehs-**tah** ehs-treh-**nyeeh**-doh (dah)?

Does he / she have vomiting?

¿Tiene vómito?
Tee-eh-neh **boh**-mee-toh?

Does he / she have decreased appetite?

¿Tiene falta de apetito?
Tee-eh-neh fahl-tah deh ah-peh-**tee**-toh?

Is he / she listless?

¿Está inquieto (a)?
Ehs-**tah** een-kee-**eh** toh (tah)?

Is he / she irritable?

¿Está irritable?
Ehs-**tah** ee-ree-**tah**-bleh?

Does he / she have problems
with his / her balance?

¿Tiene problemas con su
balance?
Tee-eh-neh proh-**bleh**-mahs
kohn soo bah-**lahn**-seh?

Does he / she have school
problems?

¿Tiene problemas escolares?
Tee-eh-neh proh-**bleh**-mahs
ehs-koh-**lah**-rehs?

Does he / she have anemia?

¿Tiene anemia?
Tee-eh-neh ah-**neh**-mee-ah?

Have you had any children
who have suffered lead
poisoning?

¿Ha tenido usted algún niño
que ha sufrido de intoxicación
del plomo?
Ah teh-**nee**-doh oos-**tehd** ahl-
goon nee-nyoh **keh** ah soo-
free-doh deh een-tog-see-kah-
see-ohn dehl **ploh**-moh?

Common Terms for Lead Screening / Toxicity

I need to examine your child.

Necesito examinar a su niño
(a).
Neh-seh-**see**-toh eg-sah-mee-
nahr a soo **nee**-nyoh (nyah).

Open your mouth and say
AH.

Abre la boca y dí AH.
Ah-breh lah **boh**-kah ee dee
ah.

Walk straight.

Camine derecho.
Kah-**mee**-neh deh-**reh**-choh.

Your child needs blood tests.

Su niño (a) necesita pruebas de sangre.
Soo **nee**-nyoh (ah) neh-seh-**see**-tah **proo-eh**-bahs deh **sahn**-greh.

Your child may have lead toxicity.

Su niño (a) puede tener intoxicación de plomo.
Soo **nee**-nyoh (ah) pweh-deh teh-**nehr** een-tog-see-kah-**see-ohn** deh **ploh**-moh.

Your child is anemic.

Su niño (a) es anémico (a).
Soo **nee**-nyoh (ah) ehs ah-**neh**-mee-koh (kah).

We need to wait for the lead screening results.

Necesitamos esperar los resultados de la prueba del plomo.
Neh-seh-see-**tah**-mohs ehs-peh-**rahr** lohs reh-sool-**tah**-dohs deh lah **proo-eh**-bah dehl **ploh**-moh.

We need to admit him / her.

Necesitamos internarlo (la).
Neh-seh-see-**tah**-mohs **een**-tehr-**nahr**-loh (lah).

Your child needs medicine to detoxify him / her.

Su niño (a) necesita medicina para desintoxicarlo (la).
Soo **nee**-nyoh (ah) neh-seh-**see**-tah meh-dee-**see**-nah pah-rah dehs-een-tog-see-**kahr**-loh (lah).

Your other children need lead screening.

Sus otros hijos necesitan la prueba del plomo.
Soos oh-trohs **ee**-hohs neh-seh-**see**-tahn lah **proo-eh**-bah dehl **ploh**-moh.

Discharge Instructions for Lead Screening / Toxicity

Call your doctor to find out about the lead screening results.

Llame a su médico para saber los resultados de la prueba del plomo.
Yah-meh a soo **meh**-dee-koh pah-rah sah-**behr** lohs rhe-sool-**tah**-dohs deh lah **proo-eh**-bah dehl **ploh**-moh.

Don't use ceramic plates.

No use platos de cerámica.
Noh **oo**-seh **plah**-tohs deh seh-**rah**-mee-kah.

Don't give him herbal or home remedies.

No le dé hierbas o remedios caseros.
Noh leh deh **yehr**-bahs oh reh-**meh**-dee-ohs kah-**seh**-rohs.

Don't let the child come in contact with peeling paint.

No deje que el niño (a) esté en contacto con pintura que se está pelando.
Noh **deh**-heh keh ehl **nee**-nyoh (nyah) ehs-**teh** ehn kohn-**tahk**-toh kohn peen-**too**-rah keh seh ehs-**tah** peh-**lahn**-doh.

Return to the hospital if your child has . . .

Regrese al hospital si su niño (a) tiene . . .
Reh-**greh**-seh ahl **ohs**-pee-tahl see soo **nee**-nyoh (nyah) **tee-eh**-neh . . .

___ vomiting

___ vómito
boh-mee-toh

___ abdominal pain

___ dolor abdominal
doh-**lohr** ab-doh-mee-**nahl**

___ problems with his / her balance

___ problemas con su balance
proh-**bleh**-mahs kohn soo bah-**lahn**-seh

Rash

Erupción

Eh-roop-**see-ohn**

When did the rash start?

¿Cuándo empezó la erupción (ronchas o manchas)?
Kwahn-doh ehm-peh-**soh** lah eh-roop-**see-ohn** (**rohn**-chahs oh **mahn**-chahs)?

It's been ___ hours ___ days.

Hace ___ horas
Ah-seh   **oh**-rahs
___ días
dee-ahs

Did it start as a . . . ?

Empezó como una . . . ?
Ehm-peh-**soh koh**-moh **oo**-nah . . . ?

___ pimple

___ espinilla
ehs-pee-**nee**-yah

___ blister

___ ampolla
ahm-**poh**-yah

___ bump

___ un grano
oon **grah**-noh

___ red spot

___ mancha roja
mahn-chah **roh**-hah

Has he / she had something
like this before?

¿Ha tenido algo así antes?
Ah teh-**nee**-doh ahl-goh ah-
see ahn-tehs?

Where did the rash begin?

¿Dónde empezaron las
ronchas o manchas?
Dohn-deh ehm-peh-**sah**-rohn
lahs **rohn**-chahs oh **mahn**-
chahs?

___ Face

___ Cara
Kah-rah

___ Chest

___ Pecho
Peh-choh

___ Back

___ Espalda
Ehs-**pahl**-dah

___ legs / arms

___ Piernas / brazos
Pee-ehr-nahs / **brah**-
sohs

Does he / she have fever?

¿Tiene fiebre?
Tee-eh-neh **fee-eh**-breh?

Does he / she have itching?

¿Tiene comezón?
Tee-eh-neh koh-meh-**sohn?**

Is his / her voice hoarse?

¿Tiene la voz ronca?
Tee-eh-neh lah bohs **rhon**-
kah?

Does he / she have trouble
breathing?

¿Tiene problemas al respirar?
Tee-eh-neh proh-**bleh**-mahs
ahl rehs-pee-**rahr?**

Is there wheezing in the
chest?

¿Le chifla el pecho?
Leh **chee**-flah ehl **peh**-choh?

Is he / she taking any medication?	¿Está tomando alguna medicina? Ehs-**tah** toh-**mahn**-doh ahl-**goo**-nah meh-dee-**see**-nah?
___ Antibiotic	___ Antibiótico Ahn-tee-bee-**oh**-tee-koh
___ Other	___ Otra Oh-trah
Does he / she have a new dog or cat?	¿Tiene un nuevo perro o gato? **Tee-eh**-neh oon **nweh**-boh **peh**-rho oh **gah**-toh?
Have you used a new soap, shampoo, detergent, or lotion?	¿Ha usado un nuevo jabón, champú, detergente, o loción? Ah oo-**sah**-doh oon **nweh**-boh ha-**bohn,** cham-**poo,** deh-tehr-**hen**-teh, oh loh-**see-ohn?**
Did you give him new foods?	¿Le dió comidas nuevas? Leh dee-**oh** koh-**mee**-dahs **nweh**-bahs?
Have you changed the formula?	¿Le ha cambiado la fórmula? Leh ah kahm-bee-**ah**-doh lah **fohr**-moo-lah?
Did you give him / her Benadryl?	¿Le dió Benadryl? Leh dee-**oh** Beh-nah-dreel?
How much did you give?	¿Cuánto le dió? **Kwahn**-toh leh dee-**oh?**
Is he / she up to date on the vaccines?	¿Está al corriente con sus vacunas? Ehs-**tah** ahl koh-rhee-**ehn**-teh kohn soos bah-**koo**-nahs?

Does he / she have allergies?   ¿Tiene alérgias?
Tee-eh-neh ah-**lehr**-hee-ahs?

Common Terms for Rash

He / she has an allergic
reaction.

Él / ella tiene una reacción
alérgica.
Ehl / eh-yah **tee-eh**-neh **oo**-
nah reh-ak-**see-ohn** ah-**lehr**-
hee-kah.

He / she has a viral infection.

Él / ella tiene una infección
viral.
Ehl / eh-yah **tee-eh**-neh **oo**-
nah een-feg-**see-ohn** bee-**rahl.**

He / she has chickenpox.

Él / ella tiene varicela
(viruela).
Ehl / eh-yah **tee-eh**-neh bah-
ree-**seh**-lah (bee-roo-**eh**-lah).

He / she has the measles.

Él / ella tiene sarampión.
Ehl / eh-yah **tee-eh**-neh sah-
rahm-**pee-ohn.**

He / she has skin infection.

Él / ella tiene una infección
de la piel.
Ehl / eh-yah **tee-eh**-neh **oo**-
nah een-feg-**see-ohn** deh lah
pee-ehl.

He / she has contact
dermatitis.

Él / ella tiene dermatitis de
contacto.
Ehl / eh-yah **tee-eh**-neh dehr-
mah-**tee**-tees deh kohn-**tahk**-
toh.

Dermatitis is an inflammation of the skin.

Dermatitis es inflamación de la piel.
Dehr-mah-**tee**-tees ehs een-flah-mah-**see-ohn** deh lah pee-ehl.

Discharge Instructions for Rash

Stop using the new soap, shampoo, cream, or detergent.

Deje de usar el nuevo jabón, champú, crema, o detergente.
Deh-he deh oo-**sahr** ehl **nweh**-boh ha-**bohn,** cham-**poo, kreh**-mah, oh deh-tehr-**hen**-teh.

If allergic to an antibiotic, stop using the antibiotic.

Si es alérgico (a) a un antibiótico, deje de usar el antibiótico.
See ehs ah-**lehr**-hee-koh (ah) ah oon ahn-tee-bee-**oh**-tee-koh, deh-he deh oo-**sahr** ehl ahn-tee-bee-**oh**-tee-koh.

Give him / her Benadryl every 6 hours.

Déle Benadryl cada seis horas.
Deh-leh Beh-nah-dreel kah-dah says **oh**-rahs.

Return to the hospital if . . .

Regrese al hospital si . . .
Reh-**greh**-seh ahl **ohs**-pee-tahl see . . .

___ he / she has shortness of breath

___ él / ella tiene falta de aire
ehl / eh-yah **tee-eh**-neh fahl-tah deh **ay**-reh

___ there is wheezing in the chest

___ le chifla el pecho
leh **chee**-flah ehl **peh**-choh

___ his / her body swells up

___ se le hincha el cuerpo
seh leh **een**-chah ehl
kwehr-poh

___ the rash worsens

___ la erupción está peor
lah eh-roop-**see-ohn**
ehs-**tah** peh-**ohr**

___ he / she has fever

___ tiene fiebre
tee-eh-neh **fee-eh**-breh

Motor Vehicle
Accident

Accidente
Automovilístico

Agsee-**dehn**-teh outoh-moh-
bee-**lees**-tee-koh

When did the accident
happen?

¿Cuándo ocurrió el accidente?
Kwahn-doh oh-koo-**rhee-oh**
ehl agsee-**dehn**-teh?

___ Hours ago

Hace ___ horas
Ah-seh   **oh**-rahs

___ Days ago

___ días
dee-ahs

Where was the child seated?

¿Dónde estaba sentado el niño
/ la niña?
Dohn-deh ehs-**tah**-bah sehn-
tah-doh ehl **nee**-nyoh / lah
nee-nyah?

___ In the front

___ Enfrente
Ehn-**frehn**-teh

___ In the back

___ Detrás
Deh-**trahs**

Was he / she in a child seat?

¿Estaba en una silla de niño?
Ehs-**tah**-bah ehn **oo**-nah **see**-yah deh **nee**-nyoh?

Did he / she have a seatbelt on?

¿Tenia puesto el cinturón de seguridad?
Teh-**nee**-ah **pwehs**-toh ehl seen-too-**rohn** deh seh-goo-ree-**dad?**

Did he / she hit the head?

¿Se pegó en la cabeza?
Seh peh-**goh** ehn lah kah-**beh**-sah?

Did he / she lose consciousness?

¿Perdió el conocimiento?
Pehr-**dee**-oh ehl koh-noh-see-mee-**ehn**-toh?

Did he / she hit his / her . . . ?

¿Se pegó en . . . ?
Seh peh-**goh** ehn . . . ?

___ chest

___ el pecho
ehl **peh**-choh

___ abdomen

___ el abdomen
ehl ab-**doh**-mehn

___ arm

___ el brazo
ehl **brah**-soh

___ leg

___ la pierna
lah **pee-ehr**-nah

Has he / she vomited after the accident?

¿Ha vomitado después del accidente?
Ah boh-mee-**tah**-doh dehs-**pwehs** dehl agsee-**dehn**-teh?

Has he / she been acting normal since the accident?

¿Ha estado actuando normal desde el accidente?
Ah ehs-**tah**-doh ahk-too-**ahn**-doh nohr-**mahl** dehs-deh ehl agsee-**dehn**-teh?

How fast was your car going?

¿A qué velocidad iba su coche?
Ah **keh** beh-loh-see-**dahd** ee-bah soo **koh**-cheh?

Were you the driver?

¿Usted fué el chofer?
Oos-**tehd fweh** ehl **choh**-fehr?

Were you the passenger?

¿Usted fué el pasajero?
Oos-**tehd fweh** ehl pah-sah-**heh**-roh?

Was the car hit . . . ?

¿Fué golpeado el coche (carro) . . . ?
Fweh gohl-peh-**ah**-doh ehl **koh**-cheh (**kah**-rho) . . . ?

___ from behind

___ por detrás
pohr deh-**trahs**

___ from the side

___ por el lado
pohr ehl lah-doh

___ head on

___ de frente
deh **frehn**-teh

Did someone die in the accident?

¿Se murió alguien en el accidente?
Seh moo-ree-**oh ahl**-gee-ehn ehn ehl agsee-**dehn**-teh?

What did you crash with?

¿Con qué chocó?
Kohn **keh** choh-**koh?**

___ Another car

___ Otro carro
Oh-troh **kah**-rho

___ A truck	___ Un camión
	Oon kah-mee-**ohn**
___ A tree	___ Un árbol
	Oon **ahr**-bohl
___ A wall	___ Una pared
	Oo-nah pah-**rehd**
___ A lamp post	___ Un poste de luz
	Oon **pohs**-teh de loos

Common Terms During the Exam for MVA

He / she needs X-rays of . . .	Él / ella necesita radiografías de . . .
	Ehl / eh-yah neh-seh-**see**-tah **rah**-dee-oh-grah-**fee-ahs** deh . . .
He / she needs a CT scan.	Él / ella necesita una tomografía computada.
	Ehl / eh-yah neh-seh-**see**-tah **oo**-nah toh-moh-grah-**fee**-ah kohm-poo-**tah**-dah.
He / she has a fracture.	Él / ella tiene una fractura.
	Ehl / eh-yah **tee-eh**-neh **oo**-nah frag-**too**-rah.
He / she has a bruise.	Él / ella tiene un moretón.
	Ehl / eh-yah **tee-eh**-neh oon moh-reh-**tohn.**

Discharge Instructions for MVA

Return to the hospital if he / she has . . .	Regrese al hospital si tiene . . .
	Reh-**greh**-seh ahl **ohs**-pee-tahl see **tee-eh**-neh . . .

___ vomiting

___ vómito
boh-mee-toh

___ headache

___ dolor de cabeza
doh-**lohr** deh kah-**beh**-
sah

___ irritability

___ irritabilidad
ee-rhee-tah-bee-lee-
dahd

___ behavior change

___ cambio en su
comportamiento
kahm-bee-oh ehn soo
kohm-pohr-tah-mee-**ehn**-
toh

Laceration

Laceración

Lah-seh-rah-**see-ohn**

How long ago did he / she
get cut?

¿Hace cuánto tiempo que se
cortó?
Ah-seh **kwahn**-toh **tee-ehm**-po
keh seh kohr-**toh?**

___ Hours

___ Horas
Oh-rahs

___ Days

___ Días
Dee-ahs

What did he / she get cut
with?

¿Con qué se cortó?
Kohn **keh** seh kohr-**toh?**

___ A knife

___ Un cuchillo
Oon koo-**chee**-yhoh

___ A switch blade

___ Una navaja
Oo-nah nah-**bah**-hah

—— A broken glass

—— Un vidrio roto
Oon **bee**-dree-oh **roh**-toh

—— A broken bottle

—— Una botella rota
Oo-nah boh-**teh**-yhah
roh-tah

—— A broken mirror

—— Un espejo roto
Oon ehs-**peh**-hoh **roh**-
toh

—— Wood

—— Madera
Mah-**deh**-rah

—— Metal

—— Metal
Meh-**tahl**

Does he / she feel something
inside the wound?

¿Siente algo dentro de la
herida?
See-ehn-teh ahl-goh **dehn**-troh
deh lah eh-**ree**-dah?

Is there redness around the
wound?

¿Está rojo alrededor de la
herida?
Ehs-**tah roh**-ho ahl-rhe-deh-
dohr deh lah eh-**ree**-dah?

Does he / she have pus from
the wound?

¿Tiene pus de la herida?
Tee-eh-neh poos deh lah eh-
ree-dah?

Does he / she have pain?

¿Tiene dolor?
Tee-neh doh-**lohr?**

Does he / she have weakness
in the . . . ?

¿Tiene debilidad en . . . ?
Tee-eh-neh deh-bee-lee-**dahd**
ehn . . . ?

—— hand

—— la mano
lah **mah**-noh

___ foot

___ el pie
ehl pee-eh

___ arm

___ el brazo
ehl **brah**-soh

___ leg

___ la pierna
lah **pee-ehr**-nah

Does he / she have numbness in the . . . ?

¿Tiene entumido (a) / adormecido (a) . . . ?
Tee-eh-neh ehn-too-**mee**-doh (ah) / ah-dohr-meh-**see**-doh (ah) . . . ?

___ hand

___ la mano
lah **mah**-noh

___ foot

___ el pie
ehl pee-eh

___ arm

___ el brazo
ehl **brah**-soh

___ leg

___ la pierna
lah **pee-ehr**-nah

Is he / she up to date with the tetanus vaccine?

¿Está al corriente con la vacuna del tétano?
Ehs-**tah** ahl koh-rhee-**ehn**-teh kohn lah bah-**koo**-nah dehl **teh**-tah-noh?

Does he / she have allergies?

¿Tiene alérgias?
Tee-eh-neh ah-**lehr**-hee-ahs?

Is he / she allergic to penicillin?

¿Es alérgico (a) a la penicilina?
Ehs ah-**lehr**-hee-koh (kah) ah lah peh-nee-see-**lee**-nah?

Common Terms During the Exam for Laceration

He / she needs stitches.

Él / ella necesita suturas.
Ehl / eh-yah neh-seh-**see**-tah soo-**too**-rahs.

We are going to clean the wound.

Vamos a limpiarle la herida.
Bah-mohs ah leem-pee-**ahr**-leh lah eh-**ree**-dah.

I am going to give him / her anesthesia.

Voy a darle anestesia.
Boy ah dahr-leh ah-nehs-**teh**-see-ah.

We need to hold him / her strongly.

Necesitamos agarrarlo (la) fuerte.
Neh-seh-see-**tah**-mohs ah-gah-**rhahr**-loh (lah) **fwehr**-teh.

These sutures are (not) absorbable.

Estas suturas (no) son absorbentes.
Ehs-tahs soo-**too**-rahs (noh) sohn ab-sohr-**behn**-tehs.

He / she needs to see a plastic surgeon.

Él / ella necesita ver a un cirujano plástico.
Ehl / eh-yah neh-seh-**see**-tah vehr ah oon see-roo-**hah**-noh **plahs**-tee-koh.

Discharge Instructions for Laceration

Keep the wound clean and dry.

Mantenga la herida limpia y seca.
Mahn-**tehn**-gah lah eh-**ree**-dah **leem**-pee-ah ee **seh**-kah.

See your doctor or return
here in two days for a wound
check.

Vea a su médico o regrese
aquí en dos días para revisarle
la herida.
Beh-ah ah soo **meh**-dee-koh
oh reh-**greh**-seh ah-**kee** ehn
dohs **dee**-ahs pah-rah reh-
bee-**sahr**-leh lah eh-**ree**-da.

Return to the hospital if he /
she has . . .

Regrese al hospital si él / ella
tiene . . .
Roh greh-seh ahl **ohs**-pee-tahl
see ehl / eh-yah **tee-eh**-
neh . . .

___ fever

___ fiebre
fee-eh-breh

___ pus from the wound

___ pus de la herida
poos deh lah eh-**ree**-dah

___ redness around the
wound

___ rojo alrededor de la
herida
roh-ho ahl-rhe-deh-**dohr**
deh lah eh-**ree**-dah

___ more pain

___ más dolor
mahs doh-**lohr**

___ more swelling

___ más hinchazón
mahs een-chah-**sohn**

The stitches need to be
removed in ___ days.

Se debe de quitarle las suturas
en ___ días.
Seh deh-beh deh kee-**tahr**-leh
lahs soo-**too**-rahs ehn ___
dee-ahs.

Give him / her the antibiotic
every ___ hours.

Déle el antibiótico cada ___
horas.
Deh-leh ehl ahn-tee-bee-**oh**-
tee-koh kah-dah ___ **oh**-rahs.

Suspected Child Abuse

Sospecha de Abuso del Niño (a)

Sohs-**peh**-chah deh ah-**boo**-soh dehl **nee**-nyoh (ah)

To the guardian

What happened?

¿Qué pasó?
Keh pah-**soh?**

Did someone hit him / her?

¿Alguien le pegó?
Ahl-gee-ehn leh peh-**goh?**

Who was it?

¿Quién fué?
Kee-**ehn fweh?**

___ The mother

___ La madre
Lah **mah**-dreh

___ The father

___ El padre
Ehl **pah**-dreh

___ The mother's boyfriend

___ El novio de la madre
Ehl **noh**-bee-oh deh lah **mah**-dreh

___ The father's girlfriend

___ La novia del padre
Lah **noh**-bee-ah dehl **pah**-dreh

___ The stepfather

___ El padrastro
Ehl pah-**drahs**-troh

___ The stepmother

___ La madrastra
Lah mah-**drahs**-trah

___ The grandfather / grandmother

___ El abuelo / la abuela
Ehl ah-**bweh**-loh / lah ah-**bweh**-lah

___ A brother

___ Un hermano
Oon ehr-**mah**-noh

___ A sister

___ Una hermana
Oo-nah ehr-**mah**-nah

___ Someone in school

___ Alguien en la escuela
Ahl-gee-ehn ehn lah
ehs-**kweh**-lah

When did you notice the
bruises?

¿Cuándo notó los moretones?
Kwahn-doh noh-**toh** lohs moh-
reh-**toh**-nehs?

Did he / she fall?

¿Se cayó?
Seh kah-**yoh?**

When did he / she fall?

¿Cuándo se cayó?
Kwahn-doh seh kah-**yoh?**

___ Today

___ Hoy
Oy

___ Days ago

Hace ___ días
Ah-seh   **dee**-ahs

How did he / she fall?

¿Cómo se cayó?
Koh-moh seh kah-**yoh?**

___ While walking

___ Mientras caminaba
Mee-ehn-trahs kah-mee-
nah-bah

___ While running

___ Mientras corria
Mee-ehn-trahs koh-**rhee**-
ah

___ While playing

___ Mientras jugaba
Mee-ehn-trahs hoo-**gah**-
bah

___ From a bed

___ De la cama
Deh lah **kah**-mah

___ From the stairs

___ De las escaleras
Deh lahs ehs-kah-**leh**-
rahs

Did someone burn his / her skin?

¿Alguien le quemó la piel?
Ahl-gee-ehn leh keh-**moh** lah pee-ehl?

What was he / she burned with?

¿Con qué se quemó?
Kohn **keh** seh keh-**moh?**

—— Hot water

—— Agua caliente
Ah-gwah kah-lee-**ehn**-teh

—— Cigarettes

—— Cigarillos
See-gah-**rhee**-yohs

—— An iron

—— Una plancha
Oo-nah **plahn**-chah

—— Hot tea / coffee

—— Té / café caliente
Teh / kah-**feh** kah-lee-**ehn**-teh

What was he / she hit with?

¿Con qué le pegaron?
Kohn **keh** leh peh-**gah**-rohn?

—— The hand

—— La mano
Lah **mah**-noh

—— A stick

—— Un palo
Oon **pah**-loh

—— The fist

—— Un puño
Oon **poo**-nyoh

—— A kick

—— Una patada
Oo-nah pah-**tah**-dah

Was he / she hit in . . . ?

¿Le pegaron en . . . ?
Leh peh-**gah**-rohn ehn . . . ?

—— the hand

—— la mano
lah **mah**-noh

___ the face

___ la cara
lah **kah**-rah

___ the abdomen

___ el abdomen
ehl ab-**doh**-mehn

___ the chest

___ el pecho
ehl **peh**-choh

Did he / she tell you that someone hit him / her?

¿Le dijo a usted que alguien le pegó?
Leh dee-hoh ah oos-**tehd keh ahl**-gee-ehn leh peh-**goh?**

Have you at any time lost custody of one of your children?

¿Ha perdido usted custodia de uno de sus niños alguna vez?
Ah pehr-**dee**-doh oos-**tehd** koos-**toh**-dee-ah deh **oo**-noh deh soos **nee**-nyohs ahl-**goo**-nah behs?

How many children do you have?

¿Cuántos niños tiene?
Kwahn-tohs **nee**-nyohs **tee-eh**-neh?

How many children live with you?

¿Cuántos niños viven con usted?
Kwahn-tohs **nee**-nyohs **bee**-behn kohn oos-**tehd?**

Do you use drugs?

¿Usted usa drogas?
Oos-**tehd oo**-sah **droh**-gahs?

Do you drink alcohol?

¿Usted toma alcohol?
Oos-**tehd toh**-mah ahl-**kohl?**

Does the accused use drugs?

¿Usa drogas el acusado?
Oo-sah **droh**-gahs ehl ah-koo-**sah**-doh?

Does the accused drink alcohol?	¿Toma alcohol el acusado? **Toh**-mah ahl-**kohl** ehl ah-koo-**sah**-doh?

To the Child

Does someone hit you?	¿Alguien te pega? **Ahl**-gee-ehn teh **peh**-gah?
Who is it?	¿Quién es? Kee-**ehn** ehs?
Where did he / she hit you?	¿Dónde te pegó? **Dohn**-deh teh peh-**goh?**
Show me.	Muéstrame. **Mwehs**-trah-meh.
Did he / she hit you with the hand?	¿Te pegó con su mano? Teh peh-**goh** kohn soo **mah**-noh?
Did he / she punch you?	¿Te pegó con el puño? Teh peh-**goh** kohn ehl **poo**-nyoh?
Did he / she hit you with a stick?	¿Te pegó con un palo? Teh peh-**goh** kohn oon **pah**-loh?
Did he / she push you?	¿Te empujó? Teh ehm-poo-**hoh?**
Did he / she burn your skin?	¿Te quemó la piel? Teh keh-**moh** lah pee-ehl?
What did he / she burn you with?	¿Con qué te quemó? Kohn **keh** teh keh-**moh?**

___ Hot water

___ Agua caliente
Ah-gwah kah-lee-**ehn**-teh

___ Hot tea / coffee

___ Té / café caliente
Teh / kah-**feh** kah-lee-**ehn**-teh

___ Cigarettes

___ Cigarillos
See-gah-**rhee**-yohs

___ The iron

___ La plancha
Lah **plahn**-chah

Did he / she bite you?

¿Te mordió?
Teh mohr-dee-**oh?**

Did he / she make you sit in hot water?

¿Te hizo sentar en agua caliente?
Teh **ee**-soh sehn-**tahr** ehn **ah**-gwah kah-lee-**ehn**-teh?

Did he / she tell you not tell anyone about this?

¿Te dijo que no le dijeras nada a nadie?
Teh dee-hoh **keh** noh leh dee-**heh**-rahs nah-dah ah **nah**-dee-eh?

Common Terms During the Exam for Suspected Child Abuse

I need to take some X-rays.

Necesito sacarle radiografías.
Neh-seh-**see**-toh sah-**kahr**-leh **rah**-dee-oh-grah-**fee-ahs.**

Your child has a fracture.

Su niño (a) tiene una fractura.
Soo **nee**-nyoh (ah) **tee-eh**-neh **oo**-nah frag-**too**-rah.

Your child has been physically abused.

Su niño (a) ha sido abusado físicamente.
Soo **nee**-nyoh (ah) ah see-doh ah-boo-**sah**-doh **fee**-see-kah-mehn-teh.

I suspect physical abuse.

Yo sospecho abuso físico.
Yoh sohs-**peh**-choh ah-**boo**-soh **fee**-see-koh.

I need to report this incident to the police.

Necesito reportar este incidente a la policía.
Neh-seh-**see**-toh reh-pohr-**tahr** ehs-teh een-see-**dehn**-teh ah lah poh-lee-**see**-ah.

I need to report this incident to the Department of Children and Family Services.

Necesito reportar este incidente al Departamento de Servicios Familiares y Niños.
Neh-seh-**see**-toh reh-pohr-**tahr** ehs-teh een-see-**dehn**-teh ahl Deh-pahr-tah-**mehn**-toh deh Sehr-**bee**-see-ohs Fah-mee-lee-**ah**-rehs ee **Nee**-nyohs.

I am going to admit him / her.

Voy a internarlo (la).
Boy ah **een**-tehr-**nahr**-loh (lah).

We are taking custody of the child.

Vamos a tomar custodia del niño / niña.
Bah-mohs ah toh-**mahr** koos-**toh**-dee-ah dehl **nee**-nyoh/ **nee**-nyah.

Discharge Instructions for Suspected Child Abuse

Go make a police report.

Vaya a hacer un reporte con la policía.
Bah-yah ah ah-**sehr** oon reh-**pohr**-teh kohn lah poh-lee-**see**-ah.

Return to the hospital if you feel that you or the child are in danger.

Regrese al hospital si siente que usted o el niño (a) está en peligro.
Reh-**greh**-seh ahl **ohs**-pee-tahl see **see-ehn**-teh **keh** oos **tehd** oh ehl **nee**-nyoh (ah) ehs-**tah** ehn peh-**lee**-groh.

Return to the hospital if the child has . . .

Regrese al hospital si el niño (a) tiene . . .
Reh-**greh**-seh ahl **ohs**-pee-tahl see ehl **nee**-nyoh (ah) **tee-eh**-neh . . .

___ headache

___ dolor de cabeza
doh-**lohr** deh kah-**beh**-sah

___ vomiting

___ vómito
boh-mee-toh

___ abdominal pain

___ dolor abdominal
doh-**lohr** ab-doh-mee-**nahl**

___ shortness of breath

___ falta de aire
fahl-tah deh ay-reh

Suspected Sexual Abuse

Sospecha de Abuso Sexual

Sohs-**peh**-chah deh ah-**boo**-soh seg-soo-**ahl**

Do you suspect that someone abused your child?

¿Usted sospecha que alguien abusó a su niño (a)?
Oos-**tehd** sohs-**peh**-chah **keh** **ahl**-gee-ehn ah-boo-**soh** ah soo **nee**-nyoh (ah)?

Who do you suspect?

¿A quién sospecha?
Ah kee-**ehn** sohs-**peh**-chah?

—— The father

—— El padre
Ehl **pah**-dreh

—— The stepfather

—— El padrastro
Ehl pah-**drahs**-troh

—— The mother's boyfriend

—— El novio de la madre
Ehl **noh**-bee-oh deh lah **mah**-dreh

—— The brother

—— El hermano
Ehl ehr-**mah**-noh

—— The stepbrother

—— El hermanastro
Ehl ehr-mah-**nahs**-troh

—— A cousin

—— Un primo
Oon **pree**-moh

—— An uncle

—— Un tío
Oon **tee**-oh

—— A family friend

—— Un amigo de la familia
Oon ah-**mee**-goh deh lah fah-**mee**-lee-ah

—— A neighbor

—— Un vecino
Oon beh-**see**-noh

—— Someone in school

—— Alguien en la escuela
Ahl-gee-ehn ehn lah ehs-**kweh**-lah

Did she tell you that someone abused her?

¿Ella le dijo a usted que alguien la abusó?
Eh-yah leh dee-ho ah oos-**tehd** keh **ahl**-gee-ehn lah ah-boo-**soh**?

Did she tell you that he touched her?

¿Ella le dijo a usted que la tocó?
Eh-yah leh dee-ho ah oos-**tehd keh** lah toh-**koh?**

Did she tell you that he kissed her?

¿Ella le dijo a usted que la besó?
Eh-yah leh dee-ho ah oos-**tehd keh** lah beh-**soh?**

Did she tell you that he violated her?

¿Ella le dijo a usted que la violó?
Eh-yah leh dee-ho ah oos-**tehd keh** lah bee-oh-**loh?**

Did she tell you if he had threatened her?

¿Ella le dijo a usted si él la amenazó?
Eh-yah leh dee-ho ah oos-**tehd** see ehl lah ah-meh-nah-**soh?**

Why do you suspect that there is abuse?

¿Porqué sospecha que hay abuso?
Pohr-**keh** sohs-**peh**-chah **keh** ay ah-**boo**-soh?

Did you notice blood in her underwear?

¿Usted notó sangre en su ropa interior?
Oos-**tehd** noh-**toh sahn**-greh ehn soo **roh**-pah een-teh-ree-**ohr?**

Did you notice discharge in her underwear?

¿Usted notó deshecho en su ropa interior?
Oos-**tehd** noh-**toh** dehs-**eh**-choh ehn soo **roh**-pah een-teh-ree-**ohr?**

Is she touching her private parts?

¿Se está tocando sus partes privadas?
Seh ehs-**tah** toh-**kahn**-doh soos **pahr**-tehs pree-**bah**-dahs?

Does she insert things in her private parts?

¿Mete cosas en sus partes privadas?

Meh-teh **koh**-sahs ehn soos **pahr**-tehs pree-**bah**-dahs?

Does she behave in a sexual manner that concerns you?

¿Se comporta de manera sexual que le preocupa a usted?

Seh kohm-**pohr**-tah deh mah-**neh**-rah seg-soo-**ahl keh** leh preh-oh-**koo**-pah ah oos-**tehd?**

Does she fear being with the person that you suspect?

¿Ella tiene miedo de estar con la persona que usted sospecha?

Eh-yah **tee-eh**-neh mee-**eh**-doh deh ehs-**tahr** kohn lah pehr-**soh**-nah **keh** oos-**tehd** sohs-**peh**-chah?

Does she hide in her room when she sees that person?

¿Se esconde en su cuarto cuando ve a esa persona?

Seh ehs-**kohn**-deh ehn soo **kwahr**-toh **kwahn**-doh beh ah eh-sah pehr-**soh**-nah?

Is she eating well?

¿Está comiendo bien?

Ehs-**tah** koh-mee-**ehn**-doh bee-ehn?

Does she play as usual?

¿Juega como siempre?

Hoo-**eh**-gah **koh**-moh see-**ehm**-preh?

Does she stay by herself in her room?

¿Se queda sola en su cuarto?

Seh **keh**-dah soh-lah ehn soo **kwahr**-toh?

Is she failing school?

¿Está reprobando en la escuela?

Ehs-**tah** reh-proh-**bahn**-doh ehn lah ehs-**kweh**-lah?

Does she wet her bed?	¿Se orina en la cama? Seh oh-**ree**-nah ehn lah **kah**-mah?
Who lives with you?	¿Quién vive con usted? Kee-**ehn bee**-beh kohn oos-**tehd?**
___ Husband	___ Esposo Ehs-**poh**-soh
___ Boyfriend	___ Novio **Noh**-bee-oh
___ Sons	___ Hijos **Ee**-hohs
___ Cousins	___ Primos **Pree**-mohs
___ Friends	___ Amigos Ah-**mee**-gohs

Questions to the child

Hello.	Hola. **Oh**-lah.
My name is . . .	Mi nombre es . . . Mee **nohm**-breh ehs . . .
I am going to ask you some questions.	Voy a hacerte algunas preguntas. Boy ah ah-**sehr**-teh ahl-**goo**-nahs preh-**goon**-tahs.
Are you afraid?	¿Tienes miedo? **Tee-eh**-nehs mee-**eh**-doh?

Do not worry, no one is going to hurt you here.

No te preocupes, nadie te va a hacer daño aquí.
Noh teh preh-oh-**koo**-pehs, **nah**-dee-eh teh bah ah ah-**sehr dah**-nyoh ah-**kee.**

What is your name?

¿Cómo te llamas?
Koh-moh teh **yah**-mahs?

How old are you?

¿Cuántos años tienes?
Kwahn-tohs **ah**-nyohs **tee-eh**-nehs?

Did someone hurt you?

¿Alguien te lastimó?
Ahl-gee-ehn teh lahs-tee-**moh?**

Who?

¿Quién?
Kee-**ehn?**

What did he do to you?

¿Qué te hizo?
Keh teh **ee**-soh?

Did he kiss you?

¿Te besó?
Teh beh-**soh?**

Did he touch you where you do not like?

¿Te tocó donde no te gusta?
Teh toh-**koh dohn**-deh noh teh **goos**-tah?

Did he touch you in places where it hurts?

¿Te tocó donde te duele?
Teh toh-**koh dohn**-deh teh dweh-leh?

Did he put something in places you do not like?

¿Te metió algo en lugares donde no te gusta?
Teh meh-tee-**oh** ahl-goh ehn loo-**gah**-rehs **dohn**-deh noh teh **goos**-tah?

Did he put something in
places that hurt you?

¿Te metió algo en lugares
donde te duele?
Teh meh-tee-**oh** ahl-goh ehn
loo-**gah**-rehs **dohn**-deh teh
dweh-leh?

Did he take off your clothes?

¿Te quitó la ropa?
Teh kee-**toh** lah **roh**-pah?

Did he take off his clothes?

¿Se quitó su ropa él?
Teh kee-**toh** soo **roh**-pah ehl?

Did he tell you not to tell
anyone anything?

¿Te dijo que no le dijeras
nada a nadie?
Teh dee-hoh **keh** noh leh dee-
hee-rahs nah-dah ah **nah**-dee-
eh?

Did he threaten you?

¿Te amenazó?
Teh ah-meh-nah-**soh?**

Did he hit you?

¿Te pegó?
Teh peh-**goh?**

Did he give you money?

¿Te dió dinero?
Teh dee-**oh** dee-**neh**-roh?

Did he give you candy?

¿Te dió dulce?
Teh dee-**oh** **dool**-seh?

Did he give you a game?

¿Te dió un juego?
Teh dee-**oh** oon hoo-**eh**-goh?

Common Terms During the Exam for Suspected Sexual Abuse

I need to examine her.

Necesito examinarla.
Neh-seh-**see**-toh eg-sah-mee-
nahr-lah.

I am only going to look.

Solamente voy a ver.
Soh-lah-**mehn**-teh boy ah
behr.

I am not going to hurt you.

No te voy a hacer daño.
Noh teh boy ah ah-**sehr dah**-
nyoh.

I need to take cultures.

Necesito tomarle cultivos.
Neh-seh-**see**-toh toh-**mahr**-leh
kool-**tee**-bohs.

I do not know if she was
molested.

No sé si la han abusado.
Noh seh see lah ahn ah-boo-
sah-doh.

I think that there was abuse.

Pienso que hubo abuso.
Pee-**ehn**-soh **keh oo**-boh ah-
boo-soh.

You need to make a police
report.

Usted necesita hacer un
reporte con la policía.
Oos-**tehd** neh-seh-**see**-tah ah-
sehr oon reh-**pohr**-teh kohn
lah poh-lee-**see**-ah.

I am going to call the social
worker.

Voy a llamar a la trabajadora
social.
Boy ah yah-**mahr** ah lah trah-
bah-ha-**doh**-rah soh-see-ahl.

I need to report this to the
Department of Children and
Family Services (DCFS).

Necesito reportar esto al
Departamento de Servicios de
Familia y Niños.
Neh-seh-**see**-toh reh-pohr-**tahr**
ehs-toh ahl Deh-pahr-tah-
mehn-toh deh Sehr-**bee**-see-
ohs deh Fah-**mee**-lee-ah ee
Nee-nyohs.

We need to take custody of the child.	Necesitamos tomar custodia del niño / la niña. Neh-seh-see-**tah**-mohs toh-**mahr** koos-**toh**-dee-ah dehl **nee**-nyoh / lah **nee**-nyah.

Discharge Instructions for Suspected Sexual Abuse

Go make a police report.	Vaya a hacer un reporte a la policía. Bah-yah ah ah-**sehr** oon reh-**pohr**-teh ah lah poh-lee-**see**-ah.
Return to the hospital if the child has . . .	Regrese al hospital si la niña tiene . . . Reh-**greh**-seh ahl **ohs**-pee-tahl see lah **nee**-nayh **tee-eh**-neh . . .
___ abdominal pain	___ dolor abdominal doh-**lohr** ab-doh-mee-**nahl**
___ vaginal discharge	___ deshecho vaginal dehs-**eh**-choh bah-hee-**nahl**
___ vomiting	___ vómito **boh**-mee-toh

Infant Care

Circumcision Care

Cuidado de la Circunsición

Kwih-**dah**-doh deh lah seer-koon-see-**see-ohn**

When was he circumcised?

¿Cuándo le hicieron la circunsición?
Kwahn-doh leh ee-see-**eh**-rohn lah seer-koon-see-**see-ohn?**

__ Today

__ Hoy
Oy

__ Yesterday

__ Ayer
Ah-**yehr**

__ Days ago

Hace __ días
Ah-seh **dee**-ahs

Is he crying more than usual?

¿Está llorando más de lo normal?
Ehs-**tah** yoh-**rahn**-doh mahs deh loh nohr-**mahl?**

Have you changed the bandage with every diaper change?

¿Le ha cambiado el vendaje cada vez que le cambia el pañal?
Leh ah kahm-bee-**ah**-doh ehl behn-**dah**-heh **kah**-dah behs **keh** leh **kahm**-bee-ah ehl pah-**nyahl?**

Is he urinating normally?

¿Está orinando normalmente?
Ehs-**tah** oh-ree-**nahn**-doh nohr-**mahl**-mehn-teh?

Is he bleeding from the penis?

¿Está sangrando del pene?
Ehs-**tah** sahn-**grahn**-doh dehl
peh-neh?

Is there redness at the tip of
the penis?

¿Está roja la punta del pene?
Ehs-**tah roh**-hah lah **poon**-tah
dehl **peh**-neh?

Is there swelling at the tip of
the penis?

¿Tiene hinchazón en la punta
del pene?
Tee-eh-neh een-chah-**sohn**
ehn-lah **poon**-tah dehl **peh**-
neh?

Is there discharge from the
wound?

¿Tiene deshecho de la herida?
Tee-eh-neh dehs-**eh**-choh deh
lah eh-**ree**-dah?

What color is the discharge?

¿De qué color es el deshecho?
Deh **keh** koh-**lohr** ehs ehl
dehs-**eh**-choh?

___ Clear

___ Claro
Klah-roh

___ White

___ Blanco
Blahn-koh

___ Yellow

___ Amarillo
Ah-mah-**ree**-yoh

Common Terms for Circumcision

I am going to examine his
penis.

Voy a examinar su pene.
Boy ah eg-sah-mee-**nahr** soo
peh-neh.

I need to remove the dressing
/ gauze.

Necesito remover el vendaje /
la gaza.
Neh-seh-**see**-toh reh-moh-**behr**
ehl behn-**dah**-heh / la **gah**-sah.

He needs more frequent dressing changes.	Necesita cambios de vendaje más frecuentes. Neh-seh-**see**-tah **kahm**-bee-ohs deh behn-**dah**-heh mahs freh-**kwehn**-tehs.
He has an infection of his penis.	Tiene una infección del pene. **Tee-eh**-neh **oo**-nah een-feg-**see-ohn** dehl **peh**-neh.
He needs antibiotics.	Necesita antibióticos. Neh-seh-**see**-tah ahn-tee-bee-**oh**-tee-kohs.
He needs to be admitted.	Necesitamos internarlo. Neh-seh-see-**tah**-mohs **een**-tehr-**nahr**-loh.

Discharge Instructions for Circumcision

Return to the hospital if the child has . . .	Regrese al hospital si el niño tiene . . . Reh-**greh**-seh ahl **ohs**-pee-tahl see ehl **nee**-nyoh **tee-eh**-neh . . .
___ problems urinating	___ problemas orinando proh-**bleh**-mahs oh-ree-**nahn**-doh
___ persistent bleeding	___ sangrado persistente sahn-**grah**-doh pehr-sees-**tehn**-teh
___ more redness at the tip of the penis	___ más rojo en la punta del pene mahs **roh**-ho ehn lah **poon**-tah dehl **peh**-neh
___ pus from the wound	___ pus de la herida poos deh lah eh-**ree**-dah

___ fever

___ fiebre
fee-eh-breh

Diaper Rash

Erupción de Pañal
Eh-roop-**see-ohn** deh pah-**nyahl**

When did the rash begin?

¿Cuándo empezó la erupción?
Kwahn-doh ehm-peh-**soh** lah eh-roop-**see-ohn?**

___ Today

___ Hoy
Oy

___ Yesterday

___ Ayer
Ah-**yehr**

___ Days ago

Hace ___ días
Ah-seh **dee**-ahs

Does he / she have diarrhea?

¿Tiene diarrea?
Tee-eh-neh dee-ah-**rhe-ah?**

How many times a day?

¿Cuántas veces al día?
Kwahn-tahs **beh**-sehs ahl **dee**-ah?

Have many times a day do you change his / her diaper?

¿Cuántas veces al día le cambia el pañal?
Kwahn-tahs **beh**-sehs ahl **dee**-ah leh **kahm**-bee-ah ehl pah-**nyahl?**

Has he / she had diaper rash before?

¿Ha tenido erupción de pañal antes?
Ah teh-**nee**-doh eh-roop-**see-ohn** deh pah-**nyahl ahn**-tehs?

Is the diaper rash getting better?

¿Está mejorando la erupción?
Ehs-**tah** meh-hoh-**rahn**-doh lah eh-roop-**see-ohn?**

Is the diaper rash getting worse?

¿Está empeorando la erupción?
Ehs-**tah** ehm-peh-oh-**rahn**-doh lah eh-roop-**see-ohn?**

Does he / she have blisters or pus-filled sores?

¿Tiene ampollas o llagas con pus?
Tee-eh-neh ahm-**poh**-yahs oh **yah**-gahs kohn poos?

Is there discharge from the sores?

¿Tiene deshecho de las llagas?
Tee-eh-neh dehs-**eh**-choh deh lahs **yah**-gahs?

What color is the discharge?

¿De qué color es el deshecho?
Deh **keh** koh-**lohr** ehs ehl dehs-**eh**-choh?

___ Clear

___ Claro
Klah-roh

___ White

___ Blanco
Blahn-koh

___ Yellow

___ Amarillo
Ah-mah-**ree**-yoh

Is he / she urinating normally?

¿Está orinando normalmente?
Ehs-**tah** oh-ree-**nahn**-doh nohr-**mahl**-mehn-teh?

Is he / she taking antibiotics?

¿Está tomando antibióticos?
Ehs-**tah** toh-**mahn**-doh ahn-tee-bee-**oh**-tee-kohs?

Are you using medication for the rash?

¿Está usando medicina para la erupcion?
Ehs-**tah** oo-**sahn**-doh meh-dee-**see**-nah pah-rah lah eh-roop-**see**-ohn?

What is the name of the medication?

¿Cuál es el nombre de la medicina?
Kwahl ehs ehl **nohm**-breh deh lah meh-dee-**see**-nah?

Does he / she have fever?

¿Tiene fiebre?
Tee-eh-neh **fee-eh**-breh?

Common Terms for Diaper Rash

I am going to examine him / her.

Voy a examinarlo (la).
Boy ah eg-sah-mee-**nahr**-loh (lah).

Please take the diaper off.

Por favor quítele el pañal.
Pohr fah-**bohr kee**-teh-leh ehl pah-**nyahl.**

You can put the diaper back on.

Puede ponerle el pañal.
Pweh-deh poh-**nehr**-leh ehl pah-**nyahl.**

He / she needs more frequent diaper changes.

Necesita cambios de pañal más frecuentes.
Neh-seh-**see**-tah **kahm**-bee-ohs deh pah-**nyahl** mahs freh-**kwehn**-tehs.

He / she has a diaper rash.

Tiene una erupción de pañal.
Tee-eh-neh **oo**-nah eh-roop-**see-ohn** deh pah-**nyahl.**

He / she has an infection.

Tiene una infección.
Tee-eh-neh **oo**-nah een-feg-**see-ohn.**

He / she needs antibiotics.

Necesita antibióticos.
Neh-seh-**see**-tah ahn-tee-bee-**oh**-tee-kohs.

He / she needs a medicated cream.

Necesita una crema medicada.
Neh-seh-**see**-tah **oo**-nah **kreh**-mah meh-dee-**kah**-dah.

Discharge Instructions for Diaper Rash

Keep the area clean and dry.

Mantenga el área limpia y seca.
Mahn-**tehn**-gah ehl **ah**-reh-ah **leem**-pee-ah ee seh-kah.

Change wet or soiled diapers frequently.

Cambie frecuentemente los pañales mojados o sucios.
Kahm-bee-eh freh-kwehn-teh-**mehn**-teh lohs pah-**nyah**-lehs moh-**hah**-dohs oh **soo**-see-ohs.

Clean the area with water and let it air dry.

Limpie el área con agua y deje que se seque al aire libre.
Leem-pee-eh ehl **ah**-reh-ah kohn **ah**-gwah ee deh-heh **keh** seh **seh**-keh ahl **ay**-reh **lee**-breh.

Apply a thick layer of protective ointment or cream every ___ hours.

Aplique una capa gruesa de pomada o crema protectora cada ___ horas.
Ah-**plee**-keh **oo**-nah **kah**-pah groo-**eh**-sah deh poh-**mah**-dah oh **kreh**-mah proh-tek-**toh**-rah kah-dah ___ **oh**-rahs.

Return to the hospital if the child . . .

Regrese al hospital si el niño (a) . . . .
Reh-**greh**-seh ahl **ohs**-pee-tahl see ehl **nee**-nyoh (ah) . . .

___ has blisters or pus-filled sores

___ tiene ampollas o llagas con pus
tee-eh-neh ahm-**poh**-yahs oh **yah**-gahs kohn poos

___ has not improved in three days

___ no ha mejorado en tres días
noh ah meh-hoh-**rah**-doh ehn trehs **dee**-ahs

___ the rash is getting worse

___ está empeorando la erupción
ehs-**tah** ehm-peh-oh-**rahn**-doh lah eh-roop-**see-ohn**

Umbilical Cord Care

Cuidado del Cordón Umbilical
Kwih-**dah**-doh dehl kohr-**dohn** oom-bee-lee-**kahl**

Clean the cord three to four times a day with alcohol until the cord falls off.

Limpie el cordón umbilical (ombligo) con alcohol tres o cuatro veces al día hasta que se caiga el cordón.
Leem-pee-eh ehl kohr-**dohn** oom-bee-lee-**kahl** (ohm-**blee**-goh) trehs oh **kwah**-troh **beh**-sehs ahl **dee**-ah ahs-tah **keh** seh **kah**-ee-gah ehl kohr-**dohn.**

The cord will fall off in eight to ten days.

El cordón se caerá en ocho a diez días.
Ehl kohr-**dohn** seh kah-eh-**rah** ehn **oh**-choh ah dee-ehs **dee**-ahs.

Try to keep the diaper below the belly button until the cord has healed.

Trate de mantener el pañal debajo del ombligo hasta que sane el cordón.
Trah-teh deh mahn-teh-**nehr** ehl pah-**nyahl** deh-**bah**-hoh dehl oom-**blee**-goh ahs-tah **keh sah**-neh ehl kohr-**dohn.**

You can fold the diaper down below the belly button.

Puede doblar el pañal debajo del ombligo.
Pweh-deh doh-**blahr** ehl pah-**nyahl** deh-**bah**-hoh dehl oom-**blee**-goh.

Call the doctor if the belly button . . .

Hable con el médico si el ombligo . . .
Ah-bleh kohn soo **meh**-dee-koh see ehl ohm-**blee**-goh . . .

—— becomes red

—— se pone rojo
seh poh-neh **roh**-ho

—— continues to bleed

—— continua a sangrar
kohn-tee-**noo**-ah ah sahn-**grahr**

—— smells bad

—— huele mal
hwe-leh mahl

—— has a yellow discharge

—— tiene deshecho amarillo
tee-eh-neh dehs-**eh**-choh ah-mah-**ree**-yoh

Give him / her a sponge bath rather than a tub bath until the cord falls off.

Déle un baño de esponja y no de tina hasta que se caiga el cordón umbilical.

Deh-leh oon **bah**-nyoh deh ehs-**pohn**-hah ee noh deh tee-nah ahs-tah **keh** seh **kah**-ee-gah ehl kohr-**dohn** oom-bee-lee-**kahl.**

Appendix—Pronunciation

In Spanish, the letters are pronounced as written with the exception of the ones listed below.

a   is pronounced like a clipped *ah* as in *father*.
    For example, **aborto** (*abortion*) = (ah-**bohr**-toh)
    cama (*bed*) = (**kah**-mah)

b   sounds like *b* as in *book*.
    For example, **brazo** (*arm*) = (**brah**-soh)
    boca (*mouth*) = (**boh**-kah)

c   has a hard sound as in *come*.
    For example, **calambre** (*cramp*) = (kah-**lahm**-breh)
    cuello (*neck*) = (**kweh**-yoh)
    a soft *s* sound before an *e* or *i*
    For example, **medicina** (*medicine*) = (meh-dee-**see**-nah)
    cerebro (*brain*) = (seh-**reh**-broh)

e   sounds like *eh* as in *bed*.
    For example, **pecho** (*chest*) = (**peh**-choh)
    estómago (*stomach*) = (ehs-**toh**-mah-goh)

g   has a hard sound as in *get* if it is before *a*, *o*, or *u*.
    For example, **garganta** (*throat*) = (gahr-**gahn**-tan)
    goteo (*drip*) = (goh-**teh**-oh)
    pronounce it soft before *e* or *i*.
    For example, **vagina** (*vagina*) = (bah-**hee**-nah)
    alérgia (*allergy*) = (ah-**lehr**-hee-ah)

h   forget about this letter as it is silent.

i   is a short sound as *ee* in *meet*.
    For example, **infarto** (*infarct*) = (een-**fahr**-toh)
    infección (*infection*) = (een-feg-**see-ohn**)

j   follows the hard sound of the English *h*.
For example, **ojo** (*eye*) = (**oh**-hoh)
mejilla (*cheek*) = (meh-**hee**-yhah)

Ll   is a nasal sound pronounced like *yes* or *you*.
For example, **tobillo** (*ankle*) = (toh-**bee**-yhoh)
llaga (*sore*) = (**yah**-gah)

ñ   sounds like the English *ny* in *canyon* or *onion*.
For example, **riñón** (*kidney*) = (ree-**nyohn**)
estreñimiento (*constipation*) = (ehs-treh-nyee-mee-**ehn**-toh)

o   sounds like *oh* in low.
For example, **operación** (*operation*) = (oh-peh-rah-**see-ohn**)
orina (*urine*) = (oh-**ree**-nah)

q   has a k sound and appears before *ue* or *ui*.
For example, **quijada** (*jaw*) = (kee-**hah**-dah)
bronquitis (*bronchitis*) = (brohn-**kee**-tees)

rr   is pronounce with a hard roll like the commercial "ruffles
have ridges."
For example, **gonorrea** (*gonorrhea*) = (goh-noh-**rhe**-ah)
catarro (*cold*) = (kah-**tah**-rhoh)

v   is pronounced like the English *b*.
For example, **vesicula** (*gallbladder*) = (beh-**see**-koo-lah)
vena (*vein*) = (**beh**-nah)

y   sounds like the English *y* in *yes*.
For example, **yeso** (*cast*) = (**yeh**-soh)
sounds like *j* in *judge* if the *y* follows *n*.
For example, **inyección** (*injection*) = (een-jeg-**see-ohn**)

z   sounds like an *s* in English.
For example, **corazon** (*heart*) = (koh-rah-**sohn**)
embarazada (*pregnant*) = (ehm-bah-rah-**sah**-dah)

Index